THE
Everyday Diabetes
Cookbook

Stella Bowling

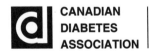
CANADIAN ASSOCIATION
DIABETES CANADIENNE
ASSOCIATION DU DIABÈTE

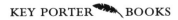
KEY PORTER BOOKS

This edition published in 1997 by Key Porter Books Limited.
First published in the United Kingdom by Grub Street, London, England.

Canadian Cataloguing in Publication Data

Bowling, Stella
    The everyday diabetes cookbook

ISBN 1-55013-755-7

1. Diabetes – Diet therapy – Recipes. I. Title.

RC662.B68   1996   641.5'6314   C96-930923-6

Canadian Diabetes Association logo and Food Choice Values and Symbols reproduced with permission of Canadian Diabetes Association.

The nutrient analysis was calculated using The Food Processor™ for Windows, v. 6.0, © 1987–1995 by ESHA Research. The analysis does not include optional ingredients or variations. Where an ingredient amount is a range, the higher number is used. Where the number of servings is a range, the lower number is used.

Key Porter Books Limited
70 The Esplanade
Toronto, Ontario
Canada M5E 1R2

Design: Jean Lightfoot Peters
Electronic formatting: Frank Zsigo
Photographs: Tim Imrie

Printed and bound in Canada

99 00   6 5 4 3 2

Contents

Acknowledgments   4

Preface   5

Recipes

    Starters   9

    Fish   25

    Vegetarian   43

    Meat and Chicken   59

    Pasta   85

    Breads   97

    Cakes and Cookies   113

    Desserts   131

    Holiday Cooking   157

Index   174

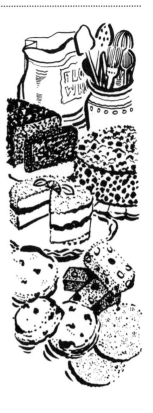

Acknowledgments

Thanks are due to Anne Dolamore of Grub Street Books in the U.K. and Sarah Trotta of Fisher Books in the U.S., for their assistance in putting this book together; to Sarah Smith, for preparing the nutritional analysis; to Katherine E. Younker, P.Dt., C.D.E., for selecting and reviewing the recipes, verifying the nutritional analysis, and assigning CDA Food Choice Values and Symbols; and to Melanie Wanless of Canadian Diabetes Association, for helping make this important book happen.

Preface

Following a healthy lifestyle means living an active life, feeling good about yourself, and eating nutritious meals. A healthy lifestyle and taking the proper medication (diabetes pills and/or insulin) are the keys to managing diabetes. *The Everyday Diabetes Cookbook* provides you with a number of interesting recipes to help add variety to your meal plan and keep you on the track to healthy eating.

It was once thought that people with diabetes had to eat "thriced"-cooked vegetables and avoid all forms of sugar. Today, people with diabetes are taught that variety, balance, and moderation are the essential components of a healthy meal plan.

Each recipe in *The Everyday Diabetes Cookbook* has Canadian Diabetes Association Food Choice Values and Symbols assigned to it. This allows you to use this book in conjunction with your *Good Health Eating Guide* meal plan.

Good Health Eating Guide

The *Good Health Eating Guide* is a system that many people with diabetes use to help them choose meals and snacks. This guide is based on *Canada's Food Guide to Healthy Eating,* with some changes made to meet the needs of people with diabetes. In particular, people with diabetes need to know the amount of carbohydrate contained in each food, along with fat and protein content.

Therefore, the *Good Health Eating Guide* breaks food into groups according to their fat, protein, and carbohydrate content. Each group has its own symbol, which makes the groups easier to use and identify. The seven groups are:

Starch Foods ▭
Fruits and Vegetables ◪
Milk ◆
Sugars ✳
Protein ⊘
Fats and Oils ▲
Extras ✚✚

Each of these groups includes many different food choices. (The word "choice" is used because of its positive meaning. You have a choice of foods from a group. The choice is yours to make!) The amount specified beside each food shows how much of that item equals one choice from the group. This way, one choice from a group can be interchanged with any other choice in the same group.

The number of food choices at any given meal will vary according to your needs. If your meal plan tells you to have two choices from a food group, you can have either two choices of two different foods in a group or two servings of one food. For example, if you have two choices from the starch group, you could have two slices of bread or one slice of bread and ½ cup (125 mL) of rice.

Your dietitian will help you plan your meals and snacks using these food groups. Your plan will tell you how many choices you can have from each of the food groups at each meal and snack.

But remember, variety is the spice of life! Choose different foods within each food group. This way, your meals and snacks will be more interesting and you can be sure to get all the nutrients you need.

You can learn about the *Good Health Eating Guide* from the following sources:

CDA Pocket Food Guide. This conveniently sized guide talks about healthy-eating principles such as variety, balance, and moderation. It also includes a tear-out section listing the food groups and their symbols for easy reference when label-reading at the grocery store.

Pocket Partner. This portable pocket/purse-size tool provides you with more information about healthy eating. It includes tips to help you with day-to-day meal planning, dining out, increasing the amount of fiber you eat, and decreasing fat in your diet. It also contains sample meal plans and much, much more.

Good Health Eating Guide Poster Pin-Up. This poster is ideal for hanging on your refrigerator door and is used by many dietitians to help develop individual meal plans for people who need one.

Good Health Eating Guide Resource. This invaluable resource comes in a convenient binder format. It discusses such topics as travel, alcohol, food labels, and vegetarian eating—all with respect to diabetes. Each of the seven food groups are listed, with an extensive (although by no means exhaustive) list of foods for each.

If you are interested in ordering any of these products, or would like more information about diabetes or Canadian Diabetes Association, contact your local Canadian Diabetes Association branch or the provincial office.

Division Offices

Alberta Division
1010-10117 Jasper Ave. NW
Edmonton, AB
T5J 1W8
Phone: (403) 423-1232
Fax: (403) 423-3322
Toll free: 1-800-563-0032

British Columbia Division
1091 West 8th Ave.
Vancouver, BC
V6H 2V3
Phone: (604) 732-1331
Fax: (604) 732-8444
Toll free: 1-800-665-6526

Manitoba Division
102-310 Broadway
Winnipeg, MB
R3C 0S6
Phone: (204) 925-3800
Fax: (204) 949-0266
Toll free: 1-800-782-0715

Nova Scotia Division
6080 Young St., Suite 101
Halifax, NS
B3K 5L2
Phone: (902) 453-4243
Fax: (902) 453-4440

Ontario Division
15 Toronto St., Suite 1001
Toronto, ON
Phone: (416) 363-3373
Fax: (416) 363-3393
Toll free: 1-800-361-1306

PEI Division
P.O. Box 133
Charlottetown, PEI
C1A 7K2
Phone: (902) 894-3005
Fax: (902) 368-1928

Saskatchewan Division
104-2301 Ave. C.N.
Saskatoon, SK
S7L 5Z5
Phone: (306) 933-1238
Fax: (306) 244-2012
Toll free: 1-800-996-4446

Affiliated with:
Association du diabète
du Québec
5635 Sherbrooke Est
Montréal, PQ
H1N 1A3
Phone: 1-800-361-3504
Fax: (514) 259-9286

New Brunswick Division
165 Regent St., Suite 3
Fredericton, NB
E3B 7B4
Phone: (506) 452-9009
Fax: (506) 455-4728
Toll free: 1-800-884-4232

Newfoundland Division
354 Water St., Suite 217
St. John's, NF
A1C 1C4
Phone: (709) 754-0953
Fax: (709) 754-0734

National Office
15 Toronto St., Suite 800
Toronto, ON
M5C 2E3
Phone: (416) 363-3373
Fax: (416) 363-3393
E-mail: info@cda-nat.org
Internet site: http://www.diabetes.ca
Toll free: 1-800-BANTING (226-8646)
Charitable registration No.: # 0160754-11

Starters

I've included a range of starters, from very light dishes, such as a fruit-filled melon, to more filling soups. The soups could also be used as a light lunch served with fresh crusty bread.

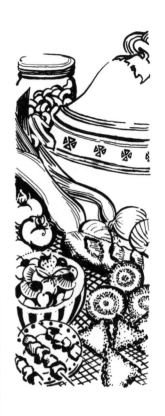

Black-Eyed Pea and Vegetable Soup

The black-eyed peas are an attractive addition, with their creamy color and small black "eye." They add a creamy flavor, too. Remember to soak the dried beans before starting this recipe.

❖ If you don't have time to soak legumes overnight, you can use the quick-soak method. Cover the legumes with plenty of boiling rather than cold water and soak only 2 to 3 hours, or bring the legumes slowly to a boil in a large pan of water. Simmer 5 minutes, cover, turn off the heat, and soak only 1 hour.

6 oz	dried black-eyed peas	175 g
1 tbsp	olive or sunflower oil	15 mL
2	medium onions, finely diced	2
1	garlic clove, crushed	1
2	carrots, peeled and finely diced	2
1	green bell pepper, finely diced	1
2	large zucchini, sliced	2
6 cups	vegetable stock	1.5 L
	Salt and freshly ground black pepper	
	Freshly chopped parsley to garnish	

Soak the beans overnight in enough cold water to cover. Drain. Heat the oil in a large saucepan over medium heat. Add the onion and cook until soft. Add the garlic, carrots, bell pepper and zucchini and cook 2 minutes. Add the stock and drained beans. Boil 10 minutes. Reduce heat, cover and simmer 50 minutes until the beans are tender. Season with salt and pepper and serve sprinkled with chopped parsley. Makes 4 to 6 servings.

PER SERVING: ¼ of recipe

2 ▧ + ½ ▨ + 1 ⊘

Calories	259
g protein	13
g carbohydrate	45
g dietary fiber	9
g fat–total	4
g saturated fat	1
mg cholesterol	0
mg sodium	174

Fresh Leek Soup with Blue Cheese

The inspiration for this recipe came from a delicious soup served at a friend's wedding reception. I decided to experiment at home to develop a similar recipe. I think the flavors of leek and blue cheese complement each other well.

1 tbsp	olive or corn oil	15 mL
1	large onion, chopped	1
1½ lb	leeks, sliced	750 g
1 tbsp	all-purpose flour	15 mL
3 cups	vegetable or chicken stock	750 mL
3 tbsp	dry white wine	50 mL
	Salt and freshly ground black pepper	
2 oz	blue cheese, crumbled	60 g
½ cup	2 percent low-fat milk	125 mL

Heat the oil in a heavy saucepan over medium heat. Add the onion and leeks and cook 5 minutes, or until softened but not colored. Stir in the flour and cook 1 minute. Remove the pan from the heat and gradually stir in the stock, wine, salt and pepper. Return the pan to the heat and bring to a boil, stirring constantly. Reduce the heat and simmer, uncovered, 20 to 30 minutes or until onion is tender.

Process in a food processor or blender until smooth. Return to the rinsed-out pan and add the cheese and milk. Heat over low heat, stirring constantly, until cheese melts. Season to taste. Serve hot with a whole-wheat roll. Makes 4 to 6 servings.

❖ Leeks are difficult to clean if you want to keep them whole. For a recipe like this, where they are to be puréed, slice the leeks lengthwise first and then across. The layers will separate and you can rinse them thoroughly in a colander under running water.

PER SERVING: ¼ of recipe

3 ▢ + 1 ▨ + 1 ◣

Calories	248
g protein	8
g carbohydrate	36
g dietary fiber	6
g fat–total	9
g saturated fat	4
mg cholesterol	13
mg sodium	392

Quick Chickpea Dip

On returning from a holiday in Crete, we held a "Greek night" for friends, and I made this dish. It is simple to make and will impress your guests, who will believe you bought it! Tahini *is a sesame paste, which is available from natural food shops, delicatessens and many supermarkets. Use small lemons—otherwise they may overpower the flavor of the dip.*

1	14-oz (398 mL) can chickpeas, drained	1
	Juice of 2 small lemons	
¼ cup	tahini paste	60 mL
3	garlic cloves, crushed	3
	Pinch cayenne pepper	
1 tbsp	chopped fresh parsley to garnish	15 mL

Place the chickpeas in a food processor or blender with the lemon juice. Blend until smooth. Add the tahini, garlic and cayenne pepper and process until blended. Spoon into a serving bowl. Sprinkle with parsley and chill before serving. Serve with warm pita bread. Makes 4 to 6 servings.

GREEK SUPPER MENU

❖ Quick Chickpea Dip (opposite) served with pita-bread fingers

❖ Light Pastitsio (page 63)

❖ Greek Salad (page 47) as a side salad

❖ Fresh fruit for dessert

PER SERVING: ⅙ of recipe

½ ▢ + ½ ▨ + 1 ◪

Calories	122
g protein	5
g carbohydrate	12
g dietary fiber	5
g fat–total	7
g saturated fat	1
mg cholesterol	0
mg sodium	143

Italian Red Bean and Pasta Soup

A filling, low-fat dish, this soup is also suitable for a lunch or light supper. You can use any pasta for it, but look for small pasta shapes, made especially for soup. They come in a variety of designs, some of which are particularly appealing to children.

2 tsp	olive or sunflower oil	10 mL
1	medium onion, finely diced	1
4	stalks celery, sliced	4
½ tsp	dried thyme	2 mL
1	7-oz can (200 mL) red kidney beans, rinsed and drained	1
1	14-oz (398 mL) can chopped tomatoes	1
2½ cups	vegetable stock	625 mL
	Salt and freshly ground black pepper	
2 oz	whole-wheat small macaroni or other pasta	60 g

Heat the oil in a large saucepan over medium heat. Add the onion, celery and thyme and cook 4 to 5 minutes, stirring occasionally. Add the beans, tomatoes, stock, salt and pepper. Bring to a boil. Reduce heat, cover and simmer 30 minutes. Add the pasta and cook 10 to 12 minutes or until the pasta is tender. Serve hot with fresh whole-wheat bread. Makes 2 to 3 servings.

❖ Kidney beans are a colorful addition to a soup. Canned ones are easy and quick to use but if you decide to use dried kidney beans, boil them 10 to 15 minutes before reducing the heat and simmering until tender. Like many beans, they contain a substance that is destroyed by boiling but can be dangerous if this is not done.

PER SERVING: ½ of recipe

2½ ▢ + 2½ ◩ + 1½ ⬕ + 1 ◣

Calories	405
g protein	17
g carbohydrate	70
g dietary fiber	9
g fat–total	8
g saturated fat	1
mg cholesterol	3
mg sodium	1758

Quick Tomato Salsa

This dish is as colorful as the Latino big-band dance music with which it shares its name. You can vary the amount of hot pepper sauce according to how spicy you like your food. Salsa is a popular Mexican dish usually served with tortilla chips.

❖ This dip is delicious with potato skins. Serve as an alternative to the tomato dip recipe given on page 19.

1	14-oz (398mL) can chopped tomatoes, drained	1
1	small onion, very finely chopped	1
1	4-oz (120 g) can green chiles, drained	1
2	garlic cloves, crushed	2
1 tbsp	white wine vinegar	15 mL
1 tbsp	tomato paste	15 mL
1 tbsp	lemon juice	15 mL
½ tsp	hot pepper sauce	2 mL
	Freshly ground black pepper	

Combine all the ingredients together in a small bowl. Cover and chill until required. Serve with tortilla chips. Makes 6 servings.

PER SERVING: ⅙ of recipe

½ ◨

Calories	26
g protein	1
g carbohydrate	6
g dietary fiber	1
g fat–total	0
g saturated fat	0
mg cholesterol	0
mg sodium	351

Chilled Summer Gazpacho

A refreshing chilled soup to serve in the summer with fresh crusty bread. Depending on the capacity of your food processor or blender, you may find it easier to process the vegetables in stages before adding the remaining ingredients to get a smoother result. Chill the soup thoroughly before serving.

2 lb	ripe tomatoes, roughly chopped	1 kg
1	large onion, roughly chopped	1
1	green bell pepper, seeded and chopped	1
1	medium cucumber, chopped	1
3 tbsp	red wine vinegar	50 mL
1 tbsp	olive oil	15 mL
2	garlic cloves, crushed	2
2½ cups	canned crushed tomatoes in purée	625 mL
	Salt and freshly ground black pepper	

Place the fresh tomatoes in a food processor or blender and blend a few seconds. Add the onion, bell pepper and cucumber and process until smooth. Add the remaining ingredients and process a few more seconds. Place in a large serving bowl, cover and chill before serving. Makes 6 to 8 servings.

❖ Serve this colorful soup with a vegetable garnish. Chop some extra or reserve a little of the tomato, bell pepper, onion and cucumber for sprinkling on top of the soup before serving. It is also delicious served with garlic croutons.

LOW-FAT GARLIC CROUTONS

❖ Cream a little soft margarine with a crushed garlic clove. Spread on a thick slice of bread. Cut into cubes and put on a baking sheet. Bake at 400°F (200°C) 10 minutes or until crisp and golden.

PER SERVING: ⅙ of recipe

2 ◨ + ½ ◣

Calories	116
g protein	4
g carbohydrate	23
g dietary fiber	5
g fat–total	3
g saturated fat	0
mg cholesterol	0
mg sodium	520

Spicy Winter Mulligatawny

For a vegetarian dish you could easily omit the chicken and use a good vegetable stock without spoiling the flavor. Serve with fresh whole-wheat bread.

❖ Mulligatawny first became popular in Britain at the end of the eighteenth century when it was brought back by employees of the East India Company who had been stationed overseas. It was changed for British cooks and is traditionally seasoned with curry powder—quite different from the spice blends that would have been used in the South-Indian original. The word comes from the Tamil words for "pepper" and "water."

2 tbsp	soft margarine	25 mL
1	large onion, finely chopped	1
2	garlic cloves, crushed	2
2	stalks celery, sliced	2
2	carrots, peeled and diced	2
1 to 2 tbsp	curry powder	15 to 25 mL
1 tbsp	all-purpose flour	15 mL
1 tbsp	tomato paste	15 mL
4 cups	chicken stock	1 L
1	medium apple, peeled, cored and diced	1
4 oz	cooked lean chicken, diced	120 g

Melt the margarine in a large saucepan over medium heat. Add the onion, garlic, celery and carrots and cook, stirring occasionally, 3 to 4 minutes or until soft. Stir in the curry powder and flour and cook, stirring, 1 minute. Stir in the tomato paste and gradually add the stock. Add the apple and bring to a boil. Reduce heat, cover and simmer 20 minutes.

Remove from the heat. Process in a food processor a few seconds to finely chop. Return to the saucepan, add the diced chicken and heat until the chicken is heated through. Serve hot. Makes 4 to 6 servings.

PER SERVING: ¼ of recipe

1½ ◪ + 1½ ◙ + ½ ▲

Calories	182
g protein	12
g carbohydrate	16
g dietary fiber	3
g fat–total	8
g saturated fat	2
mg cholesterol	16
mg sodium	905

Spicy Chicken Satay with Creamy Peanut Dip

Delicious to nibble! Don't worry if the dip looks slightly curdled after cooking. Simply allow it to cool completely, then beat in the milk.

1 lb	skinless, boneless chicken breasts	500 g
1	small onion, finely chopped	1
1	garlic clove, crushed	1
2 tbsp	light soy sauce	25 mL
2 tbsp	white wine vinegar	25 mL
1 tsp	olive or sunflower oil	5 mL
1 tsp	mild curry powder	5 mL
1 tsp	chili powder	5 mL
½ cup	natural peanut butter	125 mL
1 cup	water	250 mL
1 tbsp	skim milk	15 mL
½	small cucumber	½

Place the chicken between two sheets of waxed paper and flatten with a rolling pin. Cut into 1-inch (2.5-cm) pieces and place in a shallow container. Mix the onion and garlic with the soy sauce and vinegar. Pour over the chicken and toss well. Cover and refrigerate overnight.

Meanwhile, make the dip. Heat the oil in a small pan. Add the curry and chili powder and cook 30 to 60 seconds, stirring. Add the peanut butter and water. Simmer 2 to 3 minutes, stirring constantly, or until thickened. Allow to cool completely, then stir in the milk. Refrigerate until required. Stir before serving.

Preheat oven to 425°F (220°C). Thread the chicken onto wooden cocktail picks and place on a baking sheet. Bake 10 to 15 minutes or until cooked through, turning halfway through cooking. Brush with the marinade during the first 5 minutes of cooking only. Chill until required. Just before serving, cut the cucumber into ½-inch (1-cm) pieces and thread on to the picks with the chicken. Serve the chicken and cucumber cold with the peanut dip. Makes about 40.

PATIO PICNIC

❖ These tasty satay appetizers could also be served as a summer main course for a patio lunch or a picnic. Serve with Easy Green and Red Bean Salad (page 44), or fresh crusty bread and a green salad. This quantity serves four.

Spicy Chicken Satay

PER SERVING: ⅟₄₀ of recipe

Calories	14
g protein	2
g carbohydrate	18
g dietary fiber	0
g fat–total	0
g saturated fat	0
mg cholesterol	0
mg sodium	71

Creamy Peanut Dip

PER SERVING: ⅟₂₆ of recipe

Calories	30
g protein	1
g carbohydrate	1
g dietary fiber	0
g fat–total	3
g saturated fat	0
mg cholesterol	0
mg sodium	13

Herb and Garlic Bread

I always make my own garlic bread as I find store-bought ones disap-pointing. It is also more economical to make your own. Use a whole-wheat French loaf if possible.

❖ Suitable for freezing: Wrap well in foil. Cook from frozen in a preheated oven at 400°F (200°C) 40 to 45 minutes.

½ cup	soft margarine	125 mL
2 to 3	garlic cloves, crushed	2 to 3
2 tbsp	chopped fresh parsley	25 mL
2 tbsp	chopped fresh chives	25 mL
1	long whole-wheat French bread loaf	1

Preheat oven to 400°F (200°C). Beat together the margarine, garlic and herbs until evenly mixed. Slice the French bread at 1-inch (2.5-cm) intervals, taking care not to cut completely through the loaf. Spread each slice with the garlic mixture.

Wrap the loaf in foil and bake 20 to 25 minutes or until hot. Serve immediately. Makes 8 servings.

PER SERVING: ⅛ of recipe

2 ☐ + 2½ ▲ + 1 ⊞

Calories	262
g protein	5
g carbohydrate	32
g dietary fiber	1
g fat–total	13
g saturated fat	3
mg cholesterol	0
mg sodium	475

Crispy Potato Skins with Tomato and Yogurt Dips

Potato skins are popular as a starter and can be made easily for entertaining at home. The dips are also simple to make. Add the chili sauce carefully as it can be quite spicy!

8	small baking potatoes, about 4 oz (120 g) each	8
1 tbsp	olive oil	15 mL
	Sea salt and freshly ground black pepper	
12 oz	tomatoes, peeled and finely chopped	350 g
2	green onions, finely chopped	2
1 tbsp	hot chili sauce	15 mL
¾ cup	low-fat plain yogurt or low-fat sour cream	175 mL
2 tbsp	fresh chopped chives	25 mL

Preheat oven to 400°F (200°C). Scrub the potatoes thoroughly and dry on paper towels. Brush with the oil and sprinkle with salt. Place on a baking sheet and bake 45 to 55 minutes or until soft.

Meanwhile, make the dips. Mix the tomatoes, onions and chili sauce together and season with salt and pepper. Place in a serving bowl.

In a separate bowl, mix the yogurt and chives together and season to taste. Cover the dips and chill.

Remove the potatoes from the oven and cool slightly. Cut in half lengthwise. Scoop out the flesh, leaving a layer of potato about ½ inch (1 cm) thick on the skin. Cut each skin in half lengthwise. Place the skins on a baking sheet and bake 5 to 10 minutes or until crispy. Sprinkle with a little extra salt, if desired, and serve hot with the dips. Makes 4 to 5 servings.

Crispy Potato Skins

PER SERVING: ¼ of recipe

½ ◻

Calories	44
g protein	2
g carbohydrate	10
g dietary fiber	3
g fat–total	0
g saturated fat	0
mg cholesterol	0
mg sodium	7

Tomato Dip

PER SERVING: ¼ of recipe

½ ◻

Calories	22
g protein	1
g carbohydrate	5
g dietary fiber	1
g fat–total	0
g saturated fat	0
mg cholesterol	0
mg sodium	10

Yogurt Dip

PER SERVING: ¼ of recipe

½ ◆ Skim

Calories	24
g protein	2
g carbohydrate	3
g dietary fiber	0
g fat–total	0
g saturated fat	0
mg cholesterol	1
mg sodium	33

Hearty Winter Vegetable Soup

A nourishing soup that makes use of fresh vegetables in season. It is ideal as a low-calorie lunch, served with whole-wheat bread.

❖ Pearl barley is an excellent addition to vegetable soups. It has an interesting texture and flavor but, even more importantly, the protein it contains adds to the other vegetable proteins to make a complete protein. The body can use this type more efficiently than protein from the vegetables and grains served on their own.

1 tbsp	olive or sunflower oil	15 mL
1	large onion, finely chopped	1
1	medium rutabaga, cubed	1
2	large carrots, diced	2
1	medium turnip, diced	1
2	leeks, sliced	2
½ cup	pearl barley	125 mL
1 tsp	mixed dried herbs	5 mL
4 cups	vegetable stock	1 L
	Salt and freshly ground black pepper	
2 tbsp	chopped fresh parsley	25 mL

Heat the oil in a large saucepan over medium heat. Add the vegetables, cover and cook 5 minutes or until soft. Add the barley and cook, stirring occasionally, 2 to 3 minutes.

Stir in the herbs, stock, salt and pepper. Bring to a boil. Reduce heat, cover and simmer 45 minutes or until the vegetables are tender. Adjust seasoning and serve sprinkled with parsley. Serve with whole-wheat bread. Makes 4 servings.

PER SERVING: ¼ of recipe

1 ▢ + 2 ◪ + 1 ◮	
Calories	231
g protein	5
g carbohydrate	46
g dietary fiber	10
g fat–total	4
g saturated fat	1
mg cholesterol	0
mg sodium	199

Chilled Fruit-Filled Melon

These attractive fruit-filled melon halves make a light refreshing start to a special meal and are a good way of introducing some extra fruit into your diet.

3	Ogen, Galia or other small melons	3
2	medium grapefruits	2
1	orange	1
5 oz	frozen raspberries, defrosted and drained	150 mL
	Grated peel and juice of 1 lime	
	A little artificial sweetener (optional)	
	Sprigs of fresh mint to garnish	

❖ Ogen and Galia melons both have a green flesh. The skin of a Galia melon turns from green to a yellowish-brown when ripe. A ripe melon will yield a little at the flower end (opposite end of the stalk), but the best way to tell if a melon of this type is ripe is to smell it. Sniff for a sweet, heady, musky perfume from a ripe fruit.

Cut the melons in half and discard the seeds. Scoop out a little of the flesh from the center of each half with a melon baller and place in a bowl. Peel and segment the grapefruits and orange, saving the juice. Cut the segments in half and place in the bowl, together with the juice and raspberries. Divide the fruit among the melon halves. Sprinkle with a little lime juice, the grated peel and sweetener, if using. Refrigerate and serve chilled. Finish each half with a mint sprig. Makes 6 servings.

PER SERVING: ⅙ of recipe

3 ◪

Calories	140
g protein	3
g carbohydrate	34
g dietary fiber	5
g fat–total	1
g saturated fat	0
mg cholesterol	0
mg sodium	24

Quick and Easy Sardine Pâté

Give your heart a boost with this simple spread full of health-giving omega-3 fatty acids. Because sardines have a strong taste, use only a small amount of pâté for each cracker.

❖ For most small crackers, five provide approximately 10 g of carbohydrate. As an alternative, offer celery sticks to dip instead of crackers.

2	3¾-oz (110 mL) cans sardines in olive oil, drained and flaked	2
1	8-oz (250 g) container light cream cheese	1
	Dash of hot pepper sauce	
1 tbsp	lemon juice	15 mL
	Freshly ground black pepper	
	Chopped cucumber, red or green bell peppers or olives to garnish	

Place sardines, cream cheese, hot pepper sauce, lemon juice and black pepper in a blender or food processor and process until smooth. Cover and refrigerate until chilled. Serve spread on small crackers and garnish with a little chopped cucumber, red or green peppers or olives. Makes 10 servings.

PER SERVING: ⅟₁₀ of recipe

1 ⊘ + 1 ▲

Calories	107
g protein	7
g carbohydrate	1
g dietary fiber	0
g fat–total	8
g saturated fat	3
mg cholesterol	46
mg sodium	283

Cheese and Spinach Filo Triangles

These triangles look very impressive, yet are fairly simple to make. They look similar to samosas but, because they are baked in the oven rather than fried, they are lower in both fat and calories.

1	1-lb (500 g) package frozen chopped spinach, thawed	1
1	8-oz (250 g) container light cream cheese	1
1	garlic clove, crushed	1
¼ tsp	grated nutmeg	1 mL
	Grated peel of half a lemon	
	Salt and freshly ground black pepper	
6	sheets filo pastry, thawed, if frozen	6
¼ cup	polyunsaturated margarine, melted	60 mL

Preheat oven to 400°F (200°C). Lightly greased a large baking sheet. Cook the spinach in a saucepan over medium heat about 10 minutes, stirring occasionally. Press in a sieve to drain off any remaining water and set aside to cool. Place the cheese, garlic, nutmeg and lemon peel in a bowl. Beat in the spinach, salt and pepper and mix thoroughly. Keep the filo pastry under a damp towel while working. Brush one pastry sheet at a time with a little melted margarine and cut each sheet lengthwise into 3 pieces.

Place a heaped tspful of cheese mixture at one end. Fold the pastry over diagonally and keep folding until you reach the end. Continue until all the pastry sheets and filling have been used. Place the triangles on greased baking sheet and brush the tops with the remaining margarine. Bake 8 to 10 minutes or until golden brown. Serve hot. Makes about 24.

❖ Little nibbles like these that are easy to pick up are great for starters at a barbecue party. They can be made well in advance and just popped in the oven at the last minute. They don't compete for space on the grill, and with such tasty morsels, guests won't mind the wait while the main course cooks.

BARBECUE PARTY

❖ Cheese and Spinach Filo Triangles (opposite)

❖ Marinated Chicken and Rosemary Kebabs (page 74)

❖ Tomato and Red Onion Salad (page 48) and Herb and Garlic Bread (page 18)

❖ Chocolate and Strawberry Roll (page 115)

PER SERVING: ¹⁄₂₄ of recipe

½ ◪ + 1 ◣

Calories	61
g protein	2
g carbohydrate	4
g dietary fiber	1
g fat–total	4
g saturated fat	2
mg cholesterol	7
mg sodium	141

Watercress-and-Smoked-Salmon Roll

This makes a delicious, light start to a meal. Serve with a salad garnish and thin slices of whole-wheat bread. Watercress is very rich in vitamin C.

1	5-oz (150 g) bunch watercress	1
1	8-oz (250 g) container light cream cheese	1
1 tbsp	chopped fresh chives	15 mL
1	garlic clove, crushed	1
1 tsp	lemon juice	5 mL
	Freshly ground pepper	
8 oz	smoked salmon, cut into very thin slices	250 g
1	lemon, cut into wedges	1
	Salad greens to serve	

Reserving a few sprigs for garnish, remove the stalks from the watercress and coarsely chop remaining watercress. Place the watercress, cream cheese, chives, garlic and lemon juice in a food processor or blender and blend for a few seconds. Season liberally with pepper and process until combined. Lay the pieces of salmon on a sheet of waxed paper to form a rectangle about 12 x 8 inches (30 x 20 cm). Spread the soft cheese mixture over the salmon, then carefully roll, starting from a long side and using the paper to help you. Cover and refrigerate overnight.

Cut the salmon roll crosswise into thin slices and serve garnished with lemon wedges, watercress sprigs and salad greens. Makes 6 servings.

LATE-SUMMER-
CELEBRATION LUNCH

❖ Watercress-and-Smoked-Salmon Roll (opposite) served with thin slices of crisp whole-wheat toast

❖ Creamy Leek and Ham Tart (page 62) served with boiled new potatoes and a green salad or freshly cooked broccoli

❖ Clafouti (page 153) made with small, halved plums, if cherries are unavailable.

PER SERVING: ⅙ of recipe

1½ ⊘ + 1½ ▲ + 1 ✛✛

Calories	151
g protein	11
g carbohydrate	2
g dietary fiber	1
g fat–total	11
g saturated fat	5
mg cholesterol	35
mg sodium	594

Fish

Fish is a food we should all try to eat more frequently. Fish could almost be referred to as fast food, because it cooks in just minutes. You can purchase fish, fresh or frozen, ready to cook. The lighter in color, the milder the flavor and the less fat the fish contains. Oily fish such as mackerel, sardines and herring are particularly valuable in the diet as they contain omega-3 fatty acids, which appear to have some unique way of protecting against heart disease. Oily fish is also particularly rich in vitamins A and D.

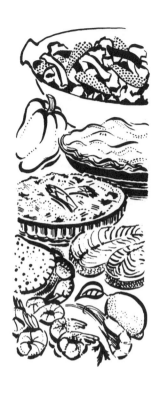

Fish with Ginger and Cilantro

A delicious and unusual way of serving fish. Serve with noodles and finely shredded vegetables.

❖ Fresh ginger root is becoming increasingly popular. It is available from the produce section in supermarkets. It keeps well in the refrigerator several days. Store in a plastic bag to prevent drying out.

4	trout, cleaned and filleted	1
1	leek, trimmed and finely sliced	1
1	medium carrot, trimmed and cut into very fine sticks	1
1	zucchini, trimmed and cut into matchstick pieces	1
1	1-inch (2.5 cm) piece ginger root, peeled and grated	1
¼ cup	chopped fresh cilantro	60 mL
	Salt and freshly ground black pepper	
2 tbsp	light soy sauce	25 mL
1	garlic clove, crushed	1
¼ cup	dry white wine	60 mL

Preheat oven to 400°F (200°C). Cut 4 rectangles of parchment paper or foil large enough to wrap around each fish. Place a fish in the center of each rectangle. Arrange the leek, carrot, zucchini, ginger and cilantro on top of each fish. Season with salt and pepper.

Mix together the soy sauce, garlic and wine in a small bowl and spoon over the fish. Fold in the edges to seal each package tightly. Place packages on a large baking sheet.

Bake 30 minutes or until the fish flakes when pierced with a fork. Makes 4 servings.

PER SERVING: ¼ of recipe

½ ◻ + 5½ ◿ + 1 ➕

Calories	292
g protein	42
g carbohydrate	8
g dietary fiber	1
g fat–total	9
g saturated fat	2
mg cholesterol	197
mg sodium	537

Baked Mushroom and Cod Crumble

Rolled oats make a nice crumble topping and are also a good source of soluble fiber, which evidence suggests can improve blood-glucose (sugar) control. The mushrooms can be replaced by peas or carrots if you like, which will also add more color to the dish.

1½ lb	cod fillets, thawed if frozen, and bones removed	750 g
1	medium onion, finely chopped	1
4 oz	mushrooms, sliced	120 g
	Freshly ground black pepper	
1	10-oz (284 mL) can condensed mushroom soup	1
1 cup	rolled oats	250 mL
¼ cup	plain whole-wheat flour	60 mL
1 tsp	dry mustard	5 mL
¼ cup	soft margarine	60 mL

Preheat oven to 375°F (190°C). Place the fish in a shallow oven-proof dish. Sprinkle the onion and mushrooms over the fish and season with pepper. Pour the soup over fish and vegetables. Place the oats, flour and mustard in a bowl and cut in the margarine until the mixture resembles bread crumbs. Sprinkle over the soup.

Bake 40 to 50 minutes or until the fish flakes when pierced with a fork. Serve with freshly cooked vegetables. Makes 4 servings.

MIDWEEK SUPPER FOR 4

❖ Quick and easy to prepare after a hard day. While the main course is in the oven, you can sit down with your feet up and unwind.

❖ Baked Mushroom and Cod Crumble (opposite) served with frozen mixed vegetables and boiled potatoes.

❖ Fresh fruit for dessert.

PER SERVING: ¼ of recipe

1 ☐ + 1 ◪ + 5 ◪ + 1 ▲

Calories	433
g protein	37
g carbohydrate	28
g dietary fiber	4
g fat–total	19
g saturated fat	4
mg cholesterol	74
mg sodium	824

Red Pepper, Basil and Tuna Pasta Salad

I often make a pasta salad for my husband to take to work as a change from sandwiches, or for us all as a lunch at the weekend. Serve with a mixed vegetable or green salad.

❖ Choose tuna packed in water rather than oil to reduce the fat content and calories. If you drain oil-packed tuna you drain away 15 to 25 percent of the health-giving omega-3 fatty acids that leach from the fish into the oil. Draining waterpacked tuna loses only about 3 percent of these beneficial fatty acids.

2	7-oz (200 mL) cans tuna packed in water, drained	2
10 oz	whole-wheat pasta twists	300 g
4 oz	green beans, trimmed and sliced	120 g
1	red bell pepper, seeded and diced	1
2 tbsp	chopped fresh basil	25 mL
1½ oz	ripe olives, halved	40 g
¼ cup	olive oil	60 mL
½ tsp	whole-grain mustard	2 mL
2 tbsp	white wine vinegar	25 mL
1	garlic clove (optional), crushed	1

Flake the tuna and place in a large serving bowl. Cook the pasta in salted boiling water according to the package instructions, 8 to 10 minutes or until al dente. Cool under cold running water and drain well.

Meanwhile, cook the green beans and bell pepper in lightly salted boiling water 2 to 3 minutes or until crisp-tender. Drain and refresh in cold water. Add to the tuna with the pasta, basil and olives. Cover and refrigerate 1 hour. Shake the remaining ingredients in a jar with a tight-fitting lid to make a dressing. Add dressing to the salad, toss to combine and serve. Makes 4 to 6 servings.

PER SERVING: ¼ of recipe

3½ ☐ + ½ ◪ + 5 ⊘

Calories	534
g protein	41
g carbohydrate	60
g dietary fiber	1
g fat–total	16
g saturated fat	2
mg cholesterol	18
mg sodium	151

Spicy Tomato and Coconut Fish Curry

This is a delicious way to serve fish because white fish absorbs the curry flavors so well. I find it spicy enough, but my husband prefers a stronger and hotter flavor, so sometimes I add an extra chile and more garam masala.

2 tbsp	olive or corn oil	25 mL
1	onion, finely chopped	1
2	garlic cloves, crushed	2
1	small green chile, seeded and finely chopped	1
1 tsp	garam masala	5 mL
1 tsp	ground cumin	5 mL
1 tbsp	tomato paste	15 mL
1 tbsp	shredded coconut	15 mL
1 cup	fish stock or chicken broth	250 mL
8 oz	peeled shrimp, thawed if frozen	250 g
1 lb	cod fillet, skinned and cubed	500 g
1 cup	frozen green peas	25 mL
	Salt and freshly ground black pepper	

Heat the oil in a large skillet or wok over medium heat and stir in the onion, garlic and chile. Cook 2 to 3 minutes, stirring constantly. Stir in the garam masala and cumin. Cook 2 minutes. Add the tomato paste, coconut and stock, and bring to a boil. Reduce the heat and add the shrimp, cod, peas, salt and pepper. Half cover and simmer 10 to 15 minutes. Serve immediately with freshly cooked brown rice. Makes 4 servings.

❖ Garam masala is a blend of spices rather than just one spice. It is available ready mixed in many Asian markets, but it is possible to blend your own to complement different dishes. Dry roast the whole spices in a pan and then grind to a powder or mix the ready ground spices. For a fish dish, ginger, coriander, cardamom, cumin and dill seeds make a nice combination.

PER SERVING: ¼ of recipe

I ◨ + 6 ▨

Calories	299
g protein	41
g carbohydrate	11
g dietary fiber	3
g fat–total	9
g saturated fat	2
mg cholesterol	172
mg sodium	596

Creamy Crab and Red Pepper Tart

Crabmeat has a meat-like texture that makes the tart very filling. You could also use tuna for this recipe as it has a similar texture.

MIDSUMMER DINNER
PARTY

❖ Spicy Chicken Satay with
Creamy Peanut Dip (page 17)
served with pita-bread fingers
or French bread

❖ Creamy Crab and Red
Pepper Tart (opposite) served
with new potatoes and a
green salad.

❖ Summer Fruit Layers (page
142) served with thin wafer
cookies

1 cup	all-purpose flour	250 mL
½ cup	whole-wheat flour	125 mL
⅓ cup	soft margarine	75 mL
3 tbsp	cold water	50 mL
1 tbsp	olive or sunflower oil	15 mL
1	small onion, finely diced	1
1	red pepper, seeded and diced	1
2	6-oz (175 g) cans crabmeat, drained, picked over and flaked	2
3	eggs, beaten	3
1 cup	2 percent low-fat milk	250 mL
	Pinch of grated nutmeg	
	Freshly ground black pepper	

Sift the flours into a bowl. Add any bran remaining in the sifter back into the bowl. Cut in the margarine until the mixture resembles fine bread crumbs. Add enough cold water to mix to a soft dough. Shape into a ball, cover and refrigerate 10 minutes.

Preheat oven to 375°F (190°C). Roll out dough on a lightly floured board to an 11-inch (28-cm) circle. Use to line a 9-inch (23-cm) tart pan. Line pastry with foil and add about 1½ cups (375 mL) dried beans. Bake 10 minutes. Remove the beans and foil and bake 5 minutes. Remove from oven and turn temperature to 350°F (180°C).

Meanwhile, heat the oil in a medium saucepan over medium heat. Add the onion and pepper and cook 5 minutes or until soft. Scatter vegetables and crabmeat over the bottom of the pastry shell.

Beat the eggs, milk, nutmeg and pepper together in a medium bowl. Pour egg mixture over vegetables and crab. Bake 40 to 50 minutes or until set and golden brown. Makes 8 servings.

PER SERVING: ⅛ of recipe

1 ▢ + ½ ◨ + 2 ⊘ + 1½ ▲

Calories	256
g protein	15
g carbohydrate	20
g dietary fiber	2
g fat–total	13
g saturated fat	3
mg cholesterol	120
mg sodium	251

Tiger Prawn Jambalaya

I find that fresh tiger prawns can be rather expensive for a weekday meal, but this makes a great informal supper dish for friends. Serve with a side salad.

2 tbsp	olive or sunflower oil	25 mL
2	large onions, finely diced	2
2	red bell peppers, seeded and finely diced	2
6	stalks celery, thinly sliced	6
1 cup	fish stock or chicken broth	250 mL
1 cup	canned crushed plum tomatoes in puree	250 mL
1 tsp	cayenne pepper	5 mL
1 tbsp	chopped fresh thyme	15 mL
2	bay leaves	2
	Salt and freshly ground black pepper	
1 cup	brown rice	250 mL
1 lb	fresh raw tiger prawns	500 g
	Chopped fresh parsley and lemon wedges to garnish	

Heat the oil in a nonstick skillet over medium-low heat. Add the onions, bell peppers and celery. Cook 5 to 10 minutes, stirring occasionally, until softened. Stir in the stock, tomatoes, cayenne pepper, thyme, bay leaves, salt and pepper. Bring to a boil, cover and simmer 30 minutes.

Meanwhile, cook the rice according to the package instructions, until just tender. Drain and keep warm.

Peel the prawns, leaving the tails on. Add the prawns to the sauce mixture and cook 3 to 5 minutes or until the prawns turn pink. Serve with the rice, garnished with parsley and lemon wedges. Makes 4 servings.

❖ Tiger prawns are very attractive with their distinctive stripes. If you buy them frozen, check if they are in a protective ice glaze, and if this is included in the weight. Sometimes it can account for almost 50 percent of the package weight.

PER SERVING: ¼ of recipe

2½ ▭ + 1 ◪ + 3½ ⊘

Calories	412
g protein	30
g carbohydrate	51
g dietary fiber	5
g fat–total	10
g saturated fat	1
mg cholesterol	0
mg sodium	483

Corn and Salmon Cakes with Yogurt-Herb Dressing

The tart, refreshing yogurt dressing combines well with these salmon cakes. Serve with a green salad and new potatoes.

❖ These salmon cakes can be frozen. Pack into a rigid container layered with pieces of waxed paper. Thaw and cook as in the recipe or, if you cook from frozen, allow 25 to 30 minutes.

1½ lb	potatoes, peeled and coarsely diced	750 g
2 tbsp	percent low-fat milk	25 mL
	Salt and freshly ground black pepper	
2	7-oz (200 mL) cans pink salmon, drained, flaked and bones removed	2
1	7-oz (200 mL) can corn with peppers, drained	1
5	green onions, finely chopped	5
	Grated peel and juice of 1 small lemon	
¼ cup	all-purpose flour	60 mL
2 oz	sesame seeds	60 g
1¼ cups	plain lowfat yogurt	300 mL
2 tbsp	chopped fresh chives	25 mL
1	4-inch (10 cm) piece cucumber, finely diced	1

RIGHT: *Italian Red Bean and Pasta Soup (page 13)*

Cook the potatoes in boiling salted water 15 minutes or until tender. Drain and mash with the milk. Season with salt and pepper. Stir in the salmon, corn, green onions, half the lemon peel and 2 tbsp (25 mL) of the lemon juice.

Sprinkle a little of the flour on a work surface. Divide the salmon mixture into 10 portions and shape into rounds with floured hands. Sprinkle both sides with sesame seeds and gently press into the flour. Cover and chill until required. Mix the yogurt, chives, remaining lemon peel and cucumber together in a small bowl. Season to taste with salt and pepper and chill until required.

Preheat oven to 375°F (190°C). Lightly grease a baking sheet. Place the salmon cakes on greased baking sheet and bake 15 to 20 minutes or until golden. Serve hot with the yogurt sauce. Makes 10 salmon cakes.

PER SERVING: ⅒ of recipe

1½ ▢ + 1½ ⬨

Calories	170
g protein	12
g carbohydrate	23
g dietary fiber	1
g fat–total	4
g saturated fat	1
mg cholesterol	20
mg sodium	363

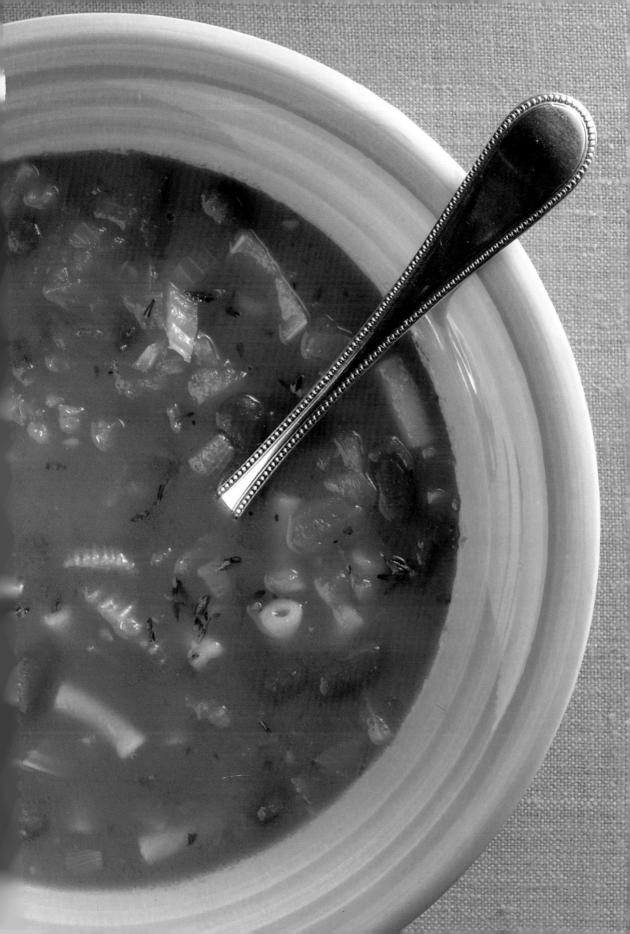

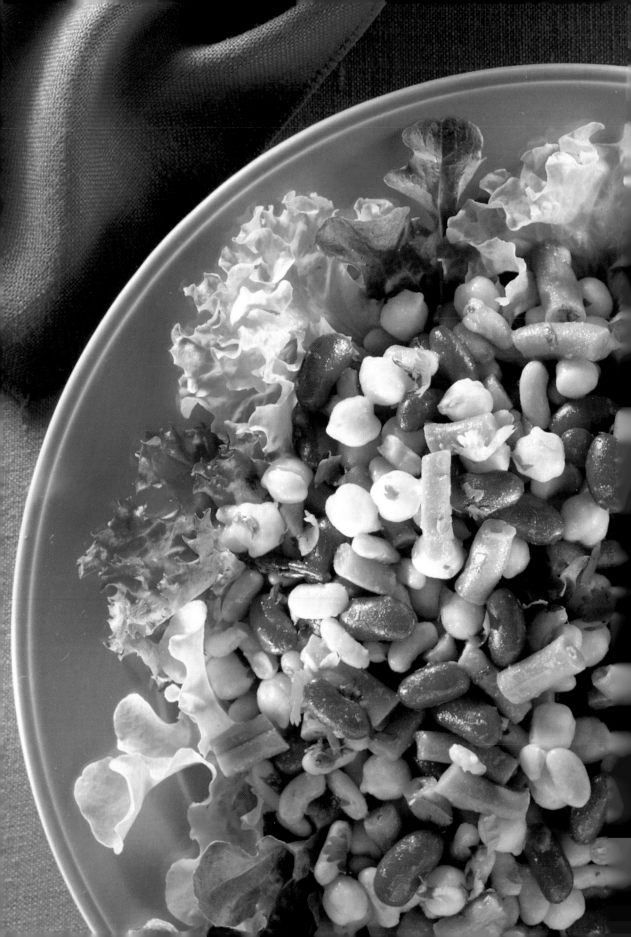

Baked Fresh Salmon and Spinach in Light Pastry

This recipe takes a little time and effort to prepare but is worth the effort. It is especially impressive to serve when entertaining.

	Grated peel and juice of ½ lemon	
	Salt and freshly ground black pepper	
1 tbsp	chopped fresh dill	15 mL
2	fresh salmon fillets, about 10 oz each	300 g
1	17-oz (475 g) package puff pastry,	1
	thawed if frozen	1
1	10-oz (300 g) package frozen chopped	1
	spinach, thawed and squeezed dry	
4 oz	light cream cheese	120 g
4 oz	brown mushrooms, sliced	120 g
1	egg, beaten	1

Combine the lemon juice and peel, black pepper and dill in a small bowl. Rub the mixture into the salmon, and place in a nonmetallic dish. Cover and marinate in the refrigerator at least 1 hour.

Preheat oven to 400°F (200°C). Keep half the pastry chilled. Roll out remaining half on a lightly floured surface to a rectangle measuring about 14 x 6 inches (35 x 15 cm). Place on a large baking sheet and prick all over with a fork. Bake 12 to 15 minutes or until golden brown and cooked through. Cool on a wire rack. Meanwhile, mix the spinach and cream cheese together and season to taste with salt and pepper. Return the cooked pastry to the baking sheet and arrange the salmon fillets on top, skinned side down. Spread the spinach mixture over the salmon, then layer with the sliced mushrooms.

Roll out the remaining pastry to 15 x 8 inches (38 x 20 cm) and place over the salmon and vegetables. Trim off any excess pastry. Slash the pastry to form a lattice pattern. Glaze all over with beaten egg. Bake 30 to 40 minutes or until the fish flakes when pierced with a fork and the pastry is puffed and golden brown. Serve hot. Makes 8 to 10 servings.

JULY 1ST DINNER

❖ For a dinner party for 8.

❖ Chilled Fruit-Filled Melon (page 21)—use 4 melons and 8 oz (250 g) raspberries for 8 people.

❖ Baked Fresh Salmon and Spinach in Light Pastry (opposite) served with new potatoes, baby carrots and snow peas

❖ Pineapple and Lemon Cheesecake (page 135)

LEFT: *Easy Green and Red Bean Salad (page 44)*

PER SERVING: ⅛ of recipe

2 ▢ + 3½ ▨ + 3½ ▲

Calories	498
g protein	28
g carbohydrate	31
g dietary fiber	2
g fat–total	29
g saturated fat	5
mg cholesterol	68
mg sodium	362

Monkfish, Tiger Prawn and Chile Stir-Fry

Monkfish lends itself well to the robust flavors of this dish. Take care when you handle fresh chiles as they can really irritate the eyes. Make sure that you wash your hands thoroughly after preparing the chiles.

❖ If you buy fresh shellfish, never freeze it. It has almost certainly already been frozen.

2	garlic cloves, crushed	2
2	tbsp light soy sauce	25 mL
4	tbsp dry sherry	60 mL
2 tbsp	lemon juice	25 mL
	Freshly ground black pepper	
1	green chile, seeded and finely chopped	1
1	bunch green onions, sliced	1
1 lb	monkfish fillet, cubed	500 g
1 tbsp	olive or sunflower oil	15 mL
4 oz	baby corn, sliced into large pieces	120 g
1	green bell pepper, seeded and sliced	1
8 oz	cooked, peeled tiger prawns	250 g
2 oz	unsalted cashew nuts	60 g

In a large bowl, mix together the garlic, soy sauce, sherry, lemon juice and pepper. Gently stir in the chile, onions and monkfish. Cover tightly and marinate in the refrigerator 2 to 4 hours, turning occasionally.

Drain the marinade and reserve. Heat the oil in a large wok or nonstick skillet over high heat. Add the monkfish mixture and stir-fry 2 to 3 minutes. Add the baby corn, bell pepper, prawns and cashews and stir-fry 1 to 2 minutes.

Pour in the reserved marinade, and boil to slightly reduce. Serve at once, with cooked brown rice or noodles. Makes 4 servings.

PER SERVING: ¼ of recipe

½ ☐ + 5 ∅ + 1 ++

Calories	317
g protein	37
g carbohydrate	11
g dietary fiber	2
g fat–total	13
g saturated fat	2
mg cholesterol	36
mg sodium	290

Zesty Lemon Fish in Packages

A quick and attractive way to serve herring. Serve with boiled new potatoes and freshly cooked vegetables.

1	medium zucchini, cut into thin strips	1
1	lemon, thinly sliced	1
1	large carrot, peeled and cut into very thin strips	1
4 oz	button mushrooms, sliced	120 g
4	6-oz (175 g) fish fillets, such as snapper or other white fish	4
¼ cup	dry white wine	60 mL
	Freshly ground black pepper	

Preheat oven to 400°F (200°C). Cut 4 rectangles of parchment paper or foil large enough to wrap around each fish fillet. Divide half the zucchini, lemon, carrot and mushrooms among the rectangles. Lay a fish fillet on top of each portion and scatter the remaining vegetables and lemon over the top. Sprinkle with the wine and season with salt and pepper. Fold in the edges to seal each package tightly. Place packages on baking sheets. Bake 10 to 15 minutes. Serve at the table in the packages for everyone to open. Makes 4 servings.

TIP

❖ Use a vegetable peeler to make very thin strips of carrot and zucchini.

PER SERVING: ¼ of recipe

6½ ☑ + 1 ++

Calories	244
g protein	46
g carbohydrate	3
g dietary fiber	1
g fat–total	3
g saturated fat	1
mg cholesterol	80
mg sodium	105

Fishermen's Crispy Filo Pie

This is perfect for company and is relatively low in fat. It is also a good source of vitamin A and folic acid. Filo pastry is a healthy option as it is low in fat. You do need to add fat by brushing it on before cooking but less than other pastries and the advantage is that you can choose the fat you use—from sinful butter to a healthful monounsaturated olive oil.

1	10-oz (300 g) package frozen chopped spinach	1
¼ cup	brown rice	60 mL
1 lb	smoked haddock fillet	500 g
1 cup	skim milk	250 mL
4 tbsp	soft margarine	60 mL
2 tbsp	all-purpose flour	25 mL
3	sheets filo pastry	3
	Salt and freshly ground black pepper	

Cook the spinach in boiling water 3 minutes. Drain well and squeeze out the excess liquid. Set aside.

Cook the rice in boiling salted water until tender. Drain well and cool.

In a covered pan, cook the fish in the milk, at just below the boiling point, about 10 minutes or until the fish flakes when pierced with a fork. Strain and reserve the cooking liquid. Flake the fish, discarding the skin and bones.

Melt 2 tbsp (25 mL) of the margarine in a saucepan. Stir in the flour and cook 1 minute. Stir in the reserved cooking liquid, bring to a boil and cook, stirring, 1 to 2 minutes or until thickened. Carefully stir in the fish. Season and set aside to cool.

Preheat oven to 400°F (200°C). Lightly grease a baking sheet. Melt the remaining margarine. Cut one sheet of filo pastry horizontally into 3 equal portions to give rectangles approximately

PER SERVING: ⅙ of recipe

❘ ▭ + 3 ⊘	
Calories	249
g protein	24
g carbohydrate	17
g dietary fiber	2
g fat–total	9
g saturated fat	2
mg cholesterol	59
mg sodium	844

7-½ x 5 inches (19 x 13 cm). Place one rectangle on greased baking sheet. Brush the pastry lightly with the melted fat. Continue layering with the remaining two rectangles. Spoon the rice onto the pastry, leaving a 1-inch (2.5-cm) border all around. Cover the rice with the spinach and then top with the fish. Cut the remaining filo pastry sheets in half and place one half on top of the filling. Brush with the fat. Layer with the remaining pastry as before. Seal the edges well and brush the top with the melted fat. Bake 20 to 30 minutes or until crisp and golden brown. Serve with boiled new potatoes and freshly cooked vegetables. Makes 6 servings.

Sweet Pepper, Baby Corn and Smoked Fish Stir-Fry

Smoked fish has a strong flavor which is not to everyone's taste. However, this stir-fry uses lots of fresh vegetables and only a small amount of fish per serving, which may persuade any reluctant fish eaters in your household.

1 tbsp	olive or sunflower oil	15 mL
1	small onion, thinly sliced	1
1	garlic clove, crushed	1
1	red bell pepper, seeded and sliced	1
1	green bell pepper, seeded and sliced	1
4 oz	baby sweet corn, sliced into large pieces	120 g
8 oz	skinned smoked fish fillet, such as mackerel, sliced	250 g
8 oz	bean sprouts	250 g
¼ cup	dry sherry or red wine	60 mL
	Freshly ground black pepper	

Heat the oil in a large skillet or wok over high heat. Add the onion and garlic and cook 2 to 3 minutes, stirring. Stir in the bell peppers and baby corn and stir-fry another 2 minutes. Stir in the smoked fish and stir-fry 4 minutes, stirring carefully.

Add the bean sprouts, sherry, salt and pepper and cook another 2 minutes. Serve immediately with brown rice or noodles. Makes 4 servings.

PER SERVING: ¼ of recipe

½ ▢ + 2 ▢ + 1½ ▲

Calories	199
g protein	14
g carbohydrate	9
g dietary fiber	3
g fat–total	12
g saturated fat	2
mg cholesterol	40
mg sodium	61

Broiled Salmon with Garlic and Peppercorns

This salmon dish is marinated in advance and takes very little time to cook, which makes it just perfect for entertaining friends, especially if you are like me and don't like missing out on the conversation while you are busy in the kitchen!

	Juice of 1 lemon	
2	garlic cloves, crushed	2
½ cup	dry white wine	125 mL
1 tbsp	crushed mixed peppercorns	15 mL
6	6 oz (175 g) salmon steaks	6
2	lemons, sliced	2

Mix the lemon juice, garlic, wine and peppercorns together in a shallow nonaluminum flameproof baking dish. Place the salmon steaks in the lemon juice mixture and turn to coat. Arrange half of the lemon slices on top of the steaks, cover and marinate in the refrigerator 2 hours or overnight.

Preheat broiler. Remove the lemon slices and broil the salmon steaks in the dish 4 to 5 minutes on each side, basting with the marinade mixture during cooking. Serve garnished with the remaining lemon slices. Makes 6 servings.

PER SERVING: ⅙ of recipe

6½ ☻

Calories	326
g protein	47
g carbohydrate	0
g dietary fiber	0
g fat–total	13
g saturated fat	3
mg cholesterol	97
mg sodium	91

Szechwan Fish Pie

Many people like the mild flavor of white fish, but this recipe shows that it is also excellent served as a spicy dish. Vary the amount of chili sauce to your taste as the quantity used is quite hot.

❖ This dish can be frozen. Thaw in the refrigerator and heat 15 to 20 minutes. Cover with foil if the pastry over-browns. Don't worry if you have used frozen fish for this dish. You can still freeze it because the fish has been cooked after thawing, thus destroying any harmful bacteria and rendering it safe to freeze again. It would, however, not be advisable to refreeze any portion that was left over after it had been reheated.

1 tbsp	olive or sunflower oil	15 mL
1½ lb	cod or other white fish fillet, skinned, bones removed and cubed	750 g
1	red bell pepper, seeded and sliced	1
1	green bell pepper, seeded and sliced	1
2	zucchinis, diced	2
2 tbsp	light soy sauce	25 mL
2 tbsp	chili sauce (or to taste)	25 mL
	Juice of 1 lemon	
1	1-inch (2.5 cm) piece ginger root, grated	1
½ cup	fish stock	125 mL
2	sheets filo pastry	2
2 tbsp	soft margarine, melted	25 mL
	Salt and freshly ground black pepper	

Preheat oven to 425°F (220°C). Heat the oil in a large saucepan, add the fish and vegetables and stir-fry 5 minutes. Spoon the mixture into a 1-quart (1-L) baking dish.

Mix together the soy sauce, chili sauce, lemon juice, ginger and stock. Season with salt and pepper and pour over the fish mixture. Brush the pastry sheets with the melted margarine and crumple over the fish. Bake 15 to 20 minutes or until crisp and golden brown. Makes 4 servings.

PER SERVING: ¼ of recipe

1½ � + 4½ ∅

Calories	249
g protein	33
g carbohydrate	17
g dietary fiber	2
g fat–total	5
g saturated fat	1
mg cholesterol	74
mg sodium	671

Flaky Salmon and Asparagus Tart

A colorful savory tart that is particularly suitable for a luncheon or buffet. Make this for a late spring treat served on the patio. Fresh asparagus is at its best in May and early June.

½ cup	all-purpose flour	125 mL
½ cup	whole-wheat flour	125 mL
¼ cup	soft margarine	60 mL
6	asparagus spears	6
1	7-oz (200 mL) can salmon, drained, flaked and bones removed	1
2	eggs	2
½ cup	skim milk	125 mL
	Salt and freshly ground black pepper	

Sift the flours into a bowl. Add any bran remaining in the sifter back into the bowl. Cut in the margarine until the mixture resembles fine bread crumbs. Add enough cold water to mix to a soft dough. Shape into a ball, cover and refrigerate 30 minutes.

Preheat oven to 400°F (200°C). Roll out dough on a lightly floured board to a 10-inch (25-cm) circle. Use to line an 8-inch (20-cm) tart pan. Blanch the asparagus in boiling salted water 5 minutes. Cool in iced water. Arrange salmon in bottom of pastry shell. Drain asparagus and arrange on top of the salmon. Beat the eggs, milk, salt and pepper together in a small bowl. Pour over the asparagus. Bake 35 to 40 minutes or until filling is set. Serve either hot or cold. Makes 6 servings.

SPRING HIGH TEA FOR 6

❖ Flaky Salmon and Asparagus Tart (opposite) served with Creamy Curried Potato Salad (page 57) and Tomato and Red Onion Salad (page 48) with fresh crusty bread

❖ Apricot-Pecan Loaf (page 102)

PER SERVING: ⅙ of recipe

1 ▢ + 1½ ⬭ + 1½ ▲

Calories	225
g protein	12
g carbohydrate	17
g dietary fiber	2
g fat–total	12
g saturated fat	2
mg cholesterol	86
mg sodium	369

Fresh Herb and Shrimp Omelet

This light and tasty omelet is ideal for summer when fresh herbs are in abundance in the garden or on your windowsill. If your green thumb fails you, many supermarkets have packages of fresh herbs these days. If all else fails, substitute dried herbs in place of fresh. You will need around 1 tsp (5 mL) of dried herbs to replace the fresh herbs in the recipe.

SUMMER LUNCH FOR 2

❖ Fresh Shrimp and Herb Omelet (opposite) served with Tomato and Red Onion Salad (page 48) and slices of warm Granary Loaf (page 110)

❖ Fresh fruit to finish

4	eggs, beaten	4
	Salt and freshly ground black pepper	
2 tbsp	skim milk	25 mL
1 tbsp	olive or sunflower oil	15 mL
3 oz	peeled cooked small shrimp, thawed if frozen	75 g
1 tbsp	fresh chopped herbs such as parsley or tarragon	15 mL

Whisk together the eggs, salt, pepper and milk. Heat the oil in a medium nonstick skillet over medium heat. Add egg mixture and cook until lightly set. Sprinkle the shrimp and herbs over the eggs and cook 2 to 3 minutes to heat through. Fold in half and serve immediately. Serve with freshly made salad and crusty bread. Makes 2 servings.

PER SERVING: ½ of recipe

3 ⊘ + 1½ ▲ + 1 ++

Calories	256
g protein	22
g carbohydrate	2
g dietary fiber	0
g fat–total	17
g saturated fat	4
mg cholesterol	508
mg sodium	496

Vegetarian

This section includes a variety of main-course recipes as well as fresh salads and vegetable side dishes to accompany meals. I have tried to include lots of legumes that contain soluble fiber, such as beans and lentils. It helps to reduce the amount of cholesterol in the blood and is a healthy addition to any meal plan. I enjoy vegetarian food and quite often choose the vegetarian option when dining out. I particularly like the spicy recipes in this section. I enjoy experimenting with different vegetables.

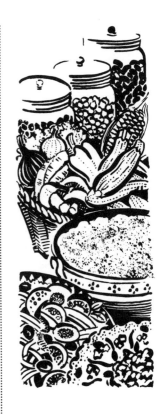

Easy Green and Red Bean Salad

I prefer to use flat-leaf parsley for the dressing. It's more distinctly flavored than curly parsley.

❖ Dressing the beans well in advance allows them to absorb all the flavors, but if you dress the salad greens too far in advance they become soft and loose their crunch. If you need to display the food in advance, such as for a buffet, you can serve the bean salad in a small dish set among the green leaves.

5 oz	green beans, trimmed and cut into small pieces	150 g
1	15-oz (425 mL) can red kidney beans, rinsed and drained	1
1	15-oz (425 mL) can flageolet beans or Great Northern beans, rinsed and drained	1
1	15-oz (425 mL) can chickpeas, rinsed and drained	1
2 tbsp	fresh parsley, chopped	25 mL
	Juice of 1 lemon	
2 tbsp	white wine vinegar	25 mL
5 tbsp	olive oil	75 mL
	Freshly ground black pepper	
	Lettuce leaves to garnish	

Lightly steam the green beans over boiling water 5 to 6 minutes or until crisp-tender. Cool in iced water and drain. Place in a large bowl with the kidney beans, flageolet beans and chickpeas and mix well.

In a jar with a tight-fitting lid, shake together the parsley, lemon juice, vinegar, olive oil and pepper. Pour over the bean mixture and toss lightly to mix. Cover and chill until served.

Just before serving, place the lettuce leaves around the edge of a large serving dish. Spoon the bean mixture over the leaves and serve. Makes 6 to 8 side-salad servings.

PER SERVING: ⅙ of recipe

2½ ▯ + 2 ⊘ + 1½ ▲

Calories	397
g protein	19
g carbohydrate	52
g dietary fiber	14
g fat–total	14
g saturated fat	2
mg cholesterol	0
mg sodium	9

Mediterranean Gougère

I often use a food processor to add the eggs to the dough mixture to obtain a smooth, glossy result. Use a slotted spoon to spoon the vegetables into the pastry ring so that the filling is not too runny.

5 tbsp	soft margarine	75 mL
1 cup	cold water	250 mL
1 cup	all-purpose flour	250 mL
½ tsp	salt	2 mL
3	eggs, beaten	3
¾ cup	shredded reduced-fat Cheddar cheese	175 mL
1 tbsp	olive or sunflower oil	15 mL
1	small onion, finely diced	1
2	garlic cloves, crushed	2
1	green bell pepper, seeded and diced	1
1	red bell pepper, seeded and diced	1
2	small zucchini, sliced	2
1	14-oz (398 mL) can chopped tomatoes, drained	1
1 tbsp	chopped fresh mixed herbs	15 mL
	Salt and freshly ground black pepper	

Preheat oven to 425°F (220°C). Place the margarine and water in a saucepan over medium heat. Bring to a boil, remove from the heat and add the flour and salt all at once. Beat well 1 to 2 minutes, or until the mixture forms a ball and leaves the sides of the pan clean. Allow to cool slightly. Gradually add the eggs, a little at a time, beating until the mixture is smooth, thick and glossy. Beat in half the cheese. Draw an 8-inch (20-cm) circle on a sheet of parchment paper and place paper on a baking sheet. Spoon or pipe the dough on to the paper to form a circle.

Bake 20 minutes. Reduce the heat to 375°F (190°C) and bake 10 minutes or until puffed and golden. Carefully remove the paper and cool on a wire rack.

❖ The cooked but unfilled pastry ring can be frozen. Cool, split horizontally and put a sheet of waxed paper between the halves. Pack into a rigid container. Thaw before filling.

PER SERVING: ⅙ of recipe

1 □ + ½ ▨ + 1 ▨ + 2½ ▲

Calories	268
g protein	10
g carbohydrate	22
g dietary fiber	2
g fat–total	16
g saturated fat	3
mg cholesterol	109
mg sodium	498

Meanwhile, heat the oil in a medium saucepan. Add the onion and garlic and cook 2 to 3 minutes or until soft, stirring occasionally. Add the bell peppers, cover and cook over low heat 5 minutes. Stir in the zucchini, tomatoes and herbs. Cook, uncovered, 15 minutes or until the vegetables are tender. Season with salt and pepper and remove from the heat.

Split the pastry ring in half horizontally. Place the bottom half on a baking sheet. With a slotted spoon, arrange vegetables in the bottom ring and cover with the top. Sprinkle with the remaining cheese and return to the oven 5 minutes to heat through. Serve immediately with new potatoes and cooked vegetables. Makes 6 servings.

Greek Salad

This is my favorite dish for a simple lunch with crusty bread. It can also be served as a side salad, where it will serve four. If you are watching calories, omit the oil and this will save a total of 200 calories.

½	head iceberg lettuce, coarsely chopped	½
½	cucumber, diced	½
2	beefsteak tomatoes, sliced	2
3 oz	feta cheese, crumbled	75 g
8	ripe Greek olives, pitted	8
2 tbsp	olive oil	25 mL
	Freshly ground black pepper	

Arrange the lettuce, cucumber, tomatoes, cheese and olives on 2 serving dishes. Drizzle with the oil and season with black pepper to taste. Makes 2 main-dish servings or 4 side-salad servings.

❖ Feta cheese is traditionally made from sheep milk but is often made from cow milk nowadays. It is usually available in the cheese section of most supermarkets and delicatessens

PER SERVING: ½ of recipe

1½ ◨ + 1½ ⊘ + 4½ ▲ + 1 ✚

Calories	375
g protein	12
g carbohydrate	23
g dietary fiber	6
g fat–total	28
g saturated fat	10
mg cholesterol	38
mg sodium	1055

Tomato and Red Onion Salad

Balsamic vinegar is an intense, rich, sweet-sour vinegar that has become very popular for cooking as well as salads. You can find it in delicatessens and most larger supermarkets.

3 tbsp	olive oil	50 mL
1 tbsp	balsamic vinegar	15 mL
	Salt and freshly ground black pepper	
1½ lb	beefsteak tomatoes, sliced	750 g
2	medium, red onions, peeled and sliced	2
	Finely chopped fresh chives to garnish	

Whisk together the oil, vinegar, salt and pepper in a large bowl. Add the tomatoes and onions and toss in the olive-oil mixture. Place in a serving bowl and let marinate in the refrigerator 30 minutes before serving. Garnish with chopped fresh chives. Makes 4 to 6 servings.

❖ Beefsteak tomatoes are extra large and sometimes irregular in shape. They are particularly good in salads because they have a firm texture. The red onion and full-flavored dressing in this salad add extra flavor.

PER SERVING: ¼ of recipe

1 ◖ + 2 ▲

Calories	146
g protein	2
g carbohydrate	13
g dietary fiber	3
g fat–total	11
g saturated fat	1
mg cholesterol	0
mg sodium	150

Light Salad Niçoise

Salad Niçoise can be quite high in fat. I've reduced the fat content by using canned tuna in water and fat-free dressing. Both products are readily available in major supermarkets. Serve with fresh crusty bread.

1	head iceberg lettuce, finely shredded	1
2	large beefsteak tomatoes, cut into wedges	2
3 oz	green beans, cooked and cooled	75 g
6	green onions, sliced	6
1	garlic clove, crushed	1
¼ cup	fat-free vinaigrette dressing	60 mL
2	7-oz (200 mL) cans tuna in water, drained	2
6	anchovy filets, drained	6
8	ripe Greek olives, pitted	8
4	hard-cooked eggs, quartered	4

Place the lettuce, tomatoes, beans and onions in a serving bowl and toss lightly together. Mix the garlic into the dressing and drizzle half of it over the contents of the bowl. Add the tuna in large chunks. Pat the anchovy filets dry on paper towels and place on top of the tuna with the olives. Drizzle with the remaining dressing and arrange the eggs on top of the salad. Serve chilled. Makes 4 servings.

❖ Vary the ingredients in this salad with sliced cucumber, strips of green pepper, tiny fresh broad beans, or for a treat add a can of drained and quartered artichoke hearts. Artichokes are high in iron and potassium, low in fat and less than 16 calories per 1 oz (25 g). The carbohydrate is negligible.

PER SERVING: ¼ of recipe

1 ◖ + 5 ◑ + 1 ++

Calories	297
g protein	37
g carbohydrate	15
g dietary fiber	4
g fat–total	10
g saturated fat	3
mg cholesterol	259
mg sodium	955

Mexican Black-Eyed Pea and Spinach Omelet

This is a great addition to a picnic basket in place of the more usual sandwiches or as a quick dish for a light supper or lunch. Serve with a side salad and fresh crusty bread.

1 tbsp	olive or sunflower oil	15 mL
1	red onion, thinly sliced	1
2	garlic cloves, crushed	2
1 tsp	ground turmeric	5 mL
1	15-oz (425 mL) can black-eyed beans, drained	1
1	10-oz (300 g) package frozen leaf spinach, thawed and squeezed dry	1
4	eggs	4
	Salt and freshly ground black pepper	

Preheat broiler. Heat the oil in a large nonstick skillet with a flame-proof handle over medium heat. Add the onion, garlic and turmeric and cook, stirring occasionally, 4 to 5 minutes. Stir in the peas and spinach.

Whisk the eggs, salt and pepper together in a medium bowl and stir into the pan to coat the other ingredients thoroughly. Cook 6 to 7 minutes or until nearly set.

Broil 2 to 3 minutes or until the omelet is set on top. Cut into wedges and serve hot or cold. Makes 2 servings.

PACK A PICNIC FOR 2

❖ Mexican Black-Eyed Pea and Spinach Omelet (opposite) served with crusty bread, cherry tomatoes and wedges of cucumber.

❖ Carrot and Banana Cake (page 114) fresh fruit

PER SERVING: ½ of recipe

2½ ☐ + ½ ◩ +
4½ ⬙ + 1 ▲

Calories	550
g protein	36
g carbohydrate	64
g dietary fiber	23
g fat–total	19
g saturated fat	4
mg cholesterol	425
mg sodium	527

Chickpea, Apricot and Cashew Pilaf

A filling dish which has a lovely combination of textures from the rice, chickpeas and cashews. It is a good source of fiber.

❖ Serve with Tomato and Red Onion Salad (page 48).

1 tbsp	olive or sunflower oil	15 mL
1	large onion, finely chopped	1
2	garlic cloves, crushed	2
1	large carrot, diced	1
1 tsp	ground cumin	5 mL
½ tsp	ground cinnamon	2 mL
1 cup	brown rice	250 mL
2½ cups	vegetable stock	625 mL
1	15-oz (425 mL) can chickpeas, drained	1
2 oz	dried apricots, chopped	60 g
3 oz	unsalted cashew nuts	75 g
2 tbsp	chopped fresh cilantro	25 mL
	Salt and freshly ground black pepper	

Heat the oil in a large nonstick skillet or saucepan over medium heat. Add the onion, garlic and carrot and cook, stirring occasionally, 5 minutes or until soft and golden. Stir in the cumin, cinnamon and rice and cook 1 minute, stirring.

Stir in the stock, bring to a boil. Reduce heat, cover and simmer 40 minutes. Stir in the chickpeas, apricots, cashews, cilantro, salt and pepper. Cook, uncovered, 5 to 10 minutes or until all the liquid has been absorbed. Serve hot. Makes 4 servings.

PER SERVING: ¼ of recipe

4½ ☐ + 1 ◧ + 1 ⊘ + 3 ◮ + 1 ⊞

Calories	570
g protein	18
g carbohydrate	90
g dietary fiber	11
g fat–total	18
g saturated fat	3
mg cholesterol	0
mg sodium	164

Flageolet Bean and Mushroom Korma

Flageolet beans were developed in Brittany in 1872 by Gabriel Chevrier. They are a green kidney bean popular in France. They are delicious just heated up as a vegetable and combine well with mushrooms to make this creamy curry. Other canned dried beans can be substituted for them.

❖ Curry paste is available in Asian markets.

1 tbsp	olive or sunflower oil	15 mL
1	red onion, chopped	1
8 oz	button mushrooms, quartered	250 g
2	garlic cloves, crushed	
1	1-inch (2.5 cm) piece ginger root, peeled and grated	1
½ cup	vegetable stock	125 mL
1	14-oz (398 mL) can flageolet beans or Great Northern beans, drained	1
1 tbsp	mild curry paste	15 mL
1 tsp	ground coriander	5 mL
	Salt and freshly ground black pepper	
¼ cup	unsalted cashew nuts	60 mL
¾ cup	low-fat plain yogurt	175 mL

Heat the oil in a saucepan over medium heat. Add the onion, mushrooms, garlic and ginger and cook 5 minutes, stirring. Add the stock, beans, curry paste, coriander, salt and pepper. Bring to a boil. Reduce heat, cover and simmer 20 minutes. Add the cashews and cook 5 minutes. Stir in the yogurt, heat through and serve immediately. Serve with cooked brown rice. Makes 2 or 3 servings.

PER SERVING: ½ of recipe

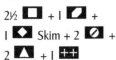

2½ ☐ + 1 ◢ +
1 ◆ Skim + 2 ⊘ +
2 ▲ + 1 ✛

Calories	464
g protein	24
g carbohydrate	59
g dietary fiber	3
g fat–total	17
g saturated fat	3
mg cholesterol	2
mg sodium	1044

Spicy Cajun Casserole

A filling casserole with a spicy punch. The heat of the chili really brings out the sweetness of the root vegetables. Serve as a main meal with fresh crusty bread, or alternatively, serve in smaller portions as a side vegetable.

❖ Suitable for freezing. Thaw completely in the refrigerator and then reheat in a saucepan. Simmer 10 minutes or until piping hot, adding a little extra water or stock if the mixture becomes too dry.

1 tbsp	olive or sunflower oil	15 mL
2	medium onions, finely diced	2
2	garlic cloves, crushed	2
3	small carrots, sliced	3
2	medium parsnips, diced	2
8 oz	button mushrooms, halved	250 g
1	green bell pepper, seeded and chopped	1
1 to 2 tsp	chili powder	5 to 10 mL
1 tbsp	tomato paste	15 mL
1½ cups	vegetable stock	375 mL
1	14-oz (398 mL) can chopped tomatoes	1
1	15-oz (425 mL) can black-eyed peas, drained	1
2 tsp	dried mixed herbs	10 mL
	A few drops hot pepper sauce	

Heat the oil in a large saucepan over medium heat. Add the onions and garlic and cook 2 to 3 minutes, stirring. Add the carrots, parsnips, mushrooms and bell pepper and cook another 5 minutes, stirring occasionally. Stir in the chili powder and tomato paste and gradually stir in the stock. Add the remaining ingredients and bring to a boil. Reduce heat, cover and simmer 40 to 50 minutes or until vegetables are tender. Serve with new potatoes or crusty bread. Makes 4 to 6 servings.

PER SERVING: ¼ of recipe

1½ ▢ + 2 ◰ + 1 ⬗ + ½ ◩

Calories	313
g protein	14
g carbohydrate	58
g dietary fiber	17
g fat–total	5
g saturated fat	1
mg cholesterol	0
mg sodium	228

Black-Eyed Pea Crumble

I make this crumb topping using a food processor. I make the bread crumbs first, add the parsley and diced cheese and then process the mixture for a few seconds.

❖ Suitable for freezing. Freeze before baking. Thaw completely in the refrigerator and then bake as directed in the recipe.

1 tbsp	olive or sunflower oil	15 mL
2	garlic cloves, crushed	2
1	leek, sliced lengthwise, rinsed well and chopped	1
3	carrots, diced	3
1	parsnip, diced	1
3	sticks celery, chopped	3
2 tsp	paprika	10 mL
1 tsp	dried oregano	5 mL
1	14-oz (398 mL) can chopped tomatoes	1
1 tbsp	tomato paste	15 mL
½ cup	vegetable stock	125 mL
	Salt and freshly ground black pepper	
1	14-oz (398 mL) can black-eyed peas, drained	1
2 cups	fresh whole-wheat bread crumbs	500 mL
2 tbsp	chopped fresh parsley	25 mL
¼ cup	finely grated vegetarian cheese	60 mL

Heat the oil in a large nonstick saucepan over medium heat. Add the garlic and leek and cook 1 to 2 minutes, stirring. Add the remaining vegetables and stir well. Stir in the paprika, oregano, tomatoes, tomato paste, stock, salt and pepper.

Bring to a boil. Reduce heat, cover and simmer 20 to 25 minutes until the vegetables are tender, but not soft. Stir in the black-eyed peas and turn into a large casserole dish.

Preheat oven to 400°F (200°C). Mix together the bread crumbs, parsley and cheese. Sprinkle over the vegetable mixture.

Bake 15 to 20 minutes or until golden brown. Serve with cooked vegetables and crusty bread or potatoes. Makes 4 servings.

PER SERVING: ¼ of recipe

2 ▭ + 1½ ◸ + 2 ⊘

Calories	342
g protein	16
g carbohydrate	61
g dietary fiber	16
g fat–total	6
g saturated fat	1
mg cholesterol	1
mg sodium	646

Lentil and Root Vegetable Hot Pot

Lentils are a good source of soluble fiber and provide the base for this filling and nutritious dish. Lentils do not require soaking before cooking as other legumes do; however, it is important that they are boiled rapidly for 10 minutes as instructed below, before adding to the hot pot.

❖ For nonvegetarians, serve with warm slices of Cheese and Bacon Bread (page 108).

8 oz	about 1 generous cup red lentils	250 mL
1 tbsp	olive or sunflower oil	15 mL
1	onion, finely diced	1
2	garlic cloves, crushed	2
2	carrots, finely diced	2
1	small rutabaga, cubed	1
3	stalks celery, sliced	3
1 cup	canned plum tomatoes in puree	250 mL
½ tsp	dried oregano	2 mL
1 cup	vegetable stock	250 mL
	Salt and freshly ground black pepper	

Cook the lentils in boiling salted water 10 minutes. Drain and rinse thoroughly.

Heat the oil in a large saucepan over medium heat. Add the onion and garlic and cook 5 minutes or until soft. Add the carrots, rutabaga and celery and cook 1 to 2 minutes, stirring occasionally. Add the lentils and the remaining ingredients and bring to a boil. Reduce heat and simmer 30 to 40 minutes or until the vegetables are tender. Ladle into warmed bowls and serve with fresh crusty bread or warmed pita bread. Makes 4 servings.

PER SERVING: ¼ of recipe

1½ ▭ + 1 ◪ + 1½ ◰

Calories	271
g protein	16
g carbohydrate	44
g dietary fiber	11
g fat–total	5
g saturated fat	1
mg cholesterol	1
mg sodium	545

Risotto Primavera

This recipe is high in complex carbohydrates and low in fat. For a nonvegetarian meal, you could add chopped cooked meat or chicken, when adding the vegetables.

1 tbsp	olive or sunflower oil	15 mL
1	onion, finely chopped	1
2	carrots, diced	2
2	medium zucchini, diced	2
4 oz	baby corn, sliced into small pieces	120 g
3	stalks celery, sliced	3
1½ cups	brown rice	375 mL
2 tsp	dried mixed herbs	10 mL
4 cups	vegetable stock	1 L
1	beefsteak tomato, peeled and chopped	1
	Salt and freshly ground black pepper	
1 tbsp	chopped fresh parsley	15 mL

Heat the oil in a heavy saucepan over medium heat. Add the onion, carrots, zucchini, baby corn and celery and cook 5 minutes or until just soft. Stir in the rice and herbs and cook 1 to 2 minutes, stirring constantly. Gradually stir in the stock, cover and simmer 45 to 50 minutes or until all the stock has been absorbed. Stir in the tomato and cook 5 minutes. Season with salt and pepper and serve hot, garnished with chopped fresh parsley. Serve with a crisp salad. Makes 4 to 6 servings.

❖ The word primavera is added to a dish to mean with fresh spring vegetables, presumably from the word primeurs, meaning early forced vegetable and fruit.

SPRING LUNCH

❖ Quick Tomato Salsa with tortilla chips (page 14)

❖ Risotto Primavera (opposite) served with a crisp salad of finely shredded spring greens.

❖ Rhubarb and Ginger Fool (page 137)

PER SERVING: ⅙ of recipe

2½ ▫ + 1½ ◪ + 1 ▲

Calories	289
g protein	7
g carbohydrate	54
g dietary fiber	4
g fat–total	5
g saturated fat	1
mg cholesterol	2
mg sodium	743

Creamy Curried Potato Salad

Keeping the skin on the potatoes retains valuable vitamins and fiber. Stir in the dressing while the potatoes are still warm so that the dressing is absorbed.

1½ lb	baby new potatoes, scrubbed	750 g
⅓ cup	low-fat sour cream	75 mL
⅓ cup	light mayonnaise	75 mL
¼ tsp	ground coriander	1 mL
¼ tsp	ground cumin	1 mL
	Salt and freshly ground black pepper	
2 tbsp	chopped fresh chives	25 mL

Cook the potatoes in boiling water until tender. Meanwhile, whisk together the sour cream, mayonnaise, coriander, cumin, salt and pepper in a large bowl. Drain the potatoes and immediately stir into the dressing. Cover and refrigerate.

Just before serving, stir in the chives. Best eaten the same day. Makes 6 to 8 servings.

❖ Serve as part of a buffet lunch with roasted chicken drumsticks, cherry tomatoes or Tomato and Red Onion Salad (page 48), and wedges of crisp lettuce. Finish with Spiced Mandarin Gâteau (page 116).

PER SERVING: ⅙ of recipe

❘ ◻ + ❘ ▲	
Calories	120
g protein	3
g carbohydrate	16
g dietary fiber	4
g fat–total	5
g saturated fat	0
mg cholesterol	4
mg sodium	245

Eastern Spiced Vegetables

I am very fond of vegetable curries and will often choose one as a vegetarian option when we have an Indian meal. This recipe can also be used as a side dish and, of course, you may vary the vegetables to suit your taste or what you have on hand.

❖ As a side dish, these spiced vegetables go very well with the Marinated Chicken and Rosemary Kebabs (page 74).

1 tbsp	olive or corn oil	15 mL
1	large onion, sliced	1
1 tbsp	curry powder	15 mL
2 tsp	chili powder	10 mL
1 tsp	ground turmeric	5 mL
1	green bell pepper, seeded and chopped	1
2	garlic cloves, crushed	2
3	small zucchini, sliced	3
2	large carrots, diced	2
4 oz	baby corn, sliced into small pieces	120 g
8 oz	cauliflower, cut into small florets	250 g
1	15-oz (425 mL) can chickpeas, drained	1
1	14-oz (398 mL) can chopped tomatoes	1
½ cup	water	125 mL
	Salt and freshly ground black pepper	

Heat the oil in a large skillet or wok over medium heat. Add the onion, curry powder, chili powder and turmeric and cook 1 to 2 minutes, stirring constantly. Stir in the remaining ingredients, bring to a boil. Reduce heat, half cover and simmer 20 minutes or until the liquid is absorbed. Serve with cooked brown rice. Makes 4 to 6 servings.

PER SERVING: ¼ of recipe

1½ □ + 1½ ◧ + 1 ⊘
+ 1 ▲

Calories	284
g protein	13
g carbohydrate	46
g dietary fiber	10
g fat–total	7
g saturated fat	1
mg cholesterol	0
mg sodium	338

Meat and Chicken

I've tried to use a variety of meats and have also included a lot of poultry recipes. The emphasis is on Mediterranean flavors and includes dishes such as kebabs and pasta dishes, but there are some traditional hearty stews and casseroles with beer or dumplings, too.

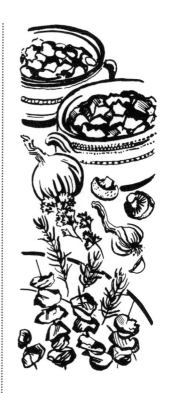

Beef Casserole with Herb Dumplings

The long, slow cooking ensures that the meat is very tender. The vegetables add rich flavor.

WINTER SUPPER FOR 4

❖ Beef Casserole with Herb Dumplings (opposite) served with new potatoes and steamed wedges of cabbage or Brussels sprouts

❖ Pears with Raspberry Sauce (page 141)

1 lb	lean beef round steak, fat removed and cubed	500 g
8 oz	rutabaga, peeled and diced	250 g
8 oz	boiling onions or shallots, peeled	250 g
5 oz	button mushrooms, halved	150 g
2	large carrots, sliced	2
1	bouquet garni	1
2 cups	beef stock	500 mL
1 tbsp	Worcestershire sauce	15 mL
	Salt and freshly ground black pepper	

Herb Dumplings

½ cup	whole-wheat flour	125 mL
½ cup	all-purpose flour	125 mL
1 tsp	baking powder	5 mL
½ tsp	salt	2 mL
2 tsp	dried Italian seasoning	10 mL
3 tbsp	vegetable oil spread	50 mL
½ cup	skim milk	125 mL

PER SERVING: ¼ of recipe

1 ▢ + 2 ◪ + 5½ ∅

Calories	481
g protein	42
g carbohydrate	41
g dietary fiber	5
g fat–total	17
g saturated fat	4
mg cholesterol	79
mg sodium	758

Preheat oven to 350°F (180°C). Place the steak, vegetables, bouquet garni, stock and Worcestershire sauce in a Dutch oven or large flameproof casserole dish. Season with salt and pepper. Bring to a boil over medium heat. Cover and bake 1 hour, stirring occasionally.

Mix together all the ingredients for the dumplings in a small bowl, adding enough to form a stiff batter. Drop 8 spoonfuls of batter onto casserole.

Bake 1 hour. Remove the bouquet garni before serving. Serve with new potatoes and cooked vegetables. Makes 4 servings.

Beef and Lentil Hot Pot

Using legumes such as lentils adds extra fiber to casserole dishes and also gives a meaty taste to the dish so that less meat is required. Lentils are low in fat and a good source of protein. Unlike most dried legumes, they do not require soaking overnight before use.

2 tbsp	all-purpose flour	25 mL
	Salt and freshly ground black pepper	
2 tsp	dried rosemary	10 mL
1¼ lb	lean beef cubes, fat removed	625 g
⅔ cup	red lentils	150 mL
1	large onion, finely diced	1
2	carrots, sliced	2
12 oz	rutabagas, diced	350 g
2½ cups	beef stock	625 mL
1½ lb	about 4 medium potatoes	750 g
1 tbsp	olive or corn oil	15 mL

Preheat oven to 325°F (160°C). Season the flour with the salt, pepper and rosemary. Toss the beef in the flour to coat evenly. Place in a Dutch oven or flameproof casserole dish.

Boil the lentils in boiling water 10 minutes. Drain, rinse and drain again. Add to the casserole dish with the onion, carrot, rutabaga and stock. Mix well. Bring to a boil over medium heat. Cover and bake 1½ hours. Peel and thinly slice the potatoes. Cover top of the casserole with potatoes and brush with oil.

Return to the oven and bake, uncovered, 1 hour or until potatoes are tender. Serve hot with cooked green vegetables. Makes 4 servings.

❖ The hot pot has had a checkered history. Originally it was a boiled mixture of ale and spirits, usually brandy, but by the middle of the nineteenth century, it had become a traditional British dish of meat and vegetables topped with potatoes. Different meats have been included over the years. For a change, try lean pork, adding a few apple slices under the potato.

PER SERVING: ¼ of recipe

½ 🔲 + ½ 🔲 + 7 🔾

Calories	715
g protein	61
g carbohydrate	70
g dietary fiber	10
g fat–total	21
g saturated fat	7
mg cholesterol	144
mg sodium	643

Creamy Leek and Ham Tart

Pastry

1 cup	whole-wheat flour	250 mL
¾ cup	all-purpose flour	175 mL
	Pinch of salt	
½ cup	margarine	125 mL
3 tbsp	water	50 mL

Leek and Ham Filling

8 oz	leeks, sliced lengthwise, rinsed well and thinly sliced crosswise	250 g
1½ cups	skim milk	375 mL
3 tbsp	all-purpose flour	50 mL
2 tbsp	margarine	25 mL
½ cup	shredded reduced-fat cheddar cheese	125 mL
2	eggs, beaten	2
2 oz	lean ham, chopped	60 g
	Freshly ground black pepper	

Sift the flours into a bowl. Add any bran remaining in the sifter back into the bowl. Cut in the margarine until the mixture resembles fine bread crumbs. Add enough cold water to mix to a soft dough. Shape into a ball, cover and refrigerate 10 minutes. Preheat oven to 400°F (200°C). Roll out dough on a lightly floured board to an 11-inch (27-cm) circle. Use to line a 9-inch (23-cm) tart pan. Line pastry with foil and add about 1½ cups (375 mL) dried beans. Bake 10 minutes. Remove the beans and foil and bake 5 minutes. Remove from oven and turn temperature to 375°F (190°C).

Cook the leeks in boiling water 10 minutes. Drain well and set aside. In a saucepan, whisk a little of the milk with the flour. Add remaining milk and margarine. Bring to a boil over medium heat, whisking constantly. Cook, whisking constantly, 1 to 2 minutes or until thickened. Remove from the heat and add a little of the hot mixture to the eggs. Return to saucepan with the cheese. Whisk together until smooth. Season with pepper. Fold in the leeks and ham. Spoon into the cooked pastry shell. Bake 35 to 40 minutes or until golden. Makes 8 servings.

PER SERVING: ⅛ of recipe

1½ ☐ + ½ ◆ Skim + 1 ⊘ + 3 ▲

Calories	296
g protein	10
g carbohydrate	27
g dietary fiber	3
g fat–total	17
g saturated fat	3
mg cholesterol	59
mg sodium	310

Light Pastitsio

This is a spicy Greek dish which I have adapted to reduce the fat content without affecting the flavor. Serve with a fresh green salad.

1 lb	extra-lean ground beef	500 g
1	large onion, finely chopped	1
2	garlic cloves, crushed	2
1 tsp	dried oregano	5 mL
1 tsp	dried thyme	5 mL
1	bay leaf	1
½ tsp	ground cinnamon	2 mL
1 tsp	ground cumin	5 mL
	Pinch of ground ginger	
	Pinch of grated nutmeg	
½ cup	dry white wine	125 mL
1	14-oz (398 mL) can chopped tomatoes	1
1 tbsp	tomato paste	15 mL
	Salt and freshly ground black pepper	
6 oz	whole-wheat pasta	175 g
2 tbsp	chopped fresh cilantro (optional)	25 mL
2 tbsp	margarine	25 mL
3 tbsp	all-purpose flour	50 mL
1½ cups	skim milk	375 mL
½ cup	shredded reduced-fat cheddar cheese	125 mL
1	egg, beaten	1

Cook beef, onion and garlic in a large nonstick pan over medium heat 5 minutes or until browned, stirring to break up beef. Stir in the herbs and spices and cook another 5 minutes, stirring occasionally.

Stir in the wine, tomatoes, tomato paste, salt and pepper. Bring to a boil, half cover and simmer 30 minutes, stirring occasionally, until the sauce is thickened and well reduced.

Meanwhile, cook the pasta in boiling, salted water until just tender. Drain and stir into the beef mixture with the chopped cilantro, if using. Spoon into a large shallow 1-quart (1-L) baking dish.

❖ Pasta is most usually thought of as an Italian dish, but before the fourth century, when Latin cookbooks record the word to mean dough, it was a food used by the Greeks and their word meant "barley porridge." Macaroni has been around since the sixteenth century. Macaroni is, in fact, a Greek word meaning "food made from barley." This Greek pasta dish is, therefore, very much an ancient specialty.

PER SERVING: ¼ of recipe

1 ☐ + 1 ◪ + ½ ◆ Skim + 5½ ⬤ + 2 ▲

Calories	558
g protein	45
g carbohydrate	29
g dietary fiber	3
g fat–total	27
g saturated fat	9
mg cholesterol	170
mg sodium	543

RIGHT: *Chicken, Spicy Sausage and Seafood Paella (page 73)*

Preheat oven to 375°F (190°C). In a saucepan, whisk a little of the milk with the flour. Add remaining milk and margarine. Bring to a boil over medium heat, whisking constantly. Cook, whisking constantly, 1 to 2 minutes or until thickened. Remove from the heat and add a little of the hot mixture to the eggs. Return to saucepan with the cheese. Whisk together until smooth.

Season with salt and pepper. Pour over the beef mixture. Bake 35 to 40 minutes or until golden brown and bubbly. Serve hot with a green salad and crusty bread, if desired. Makes 4 to 6 servings.

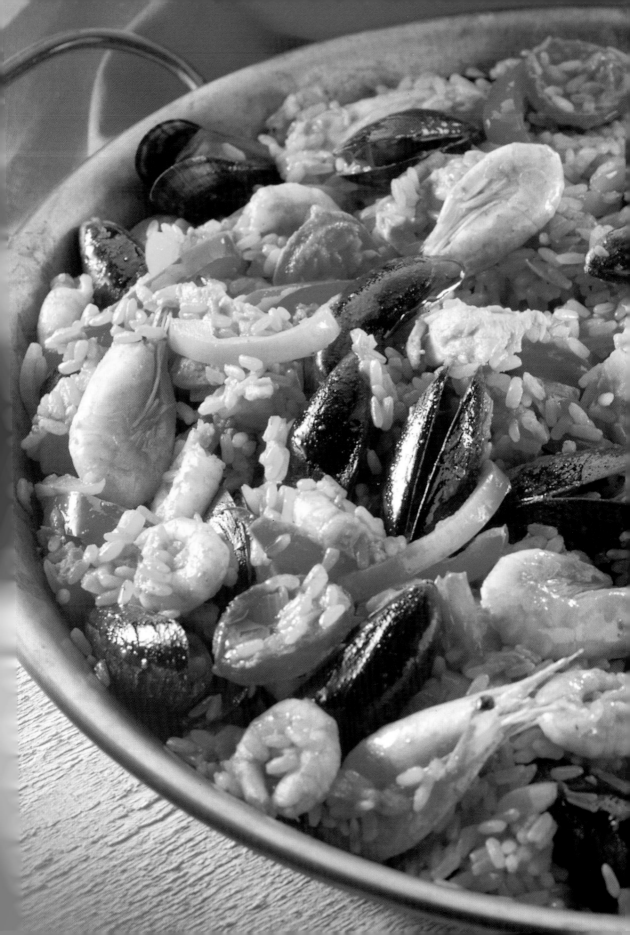

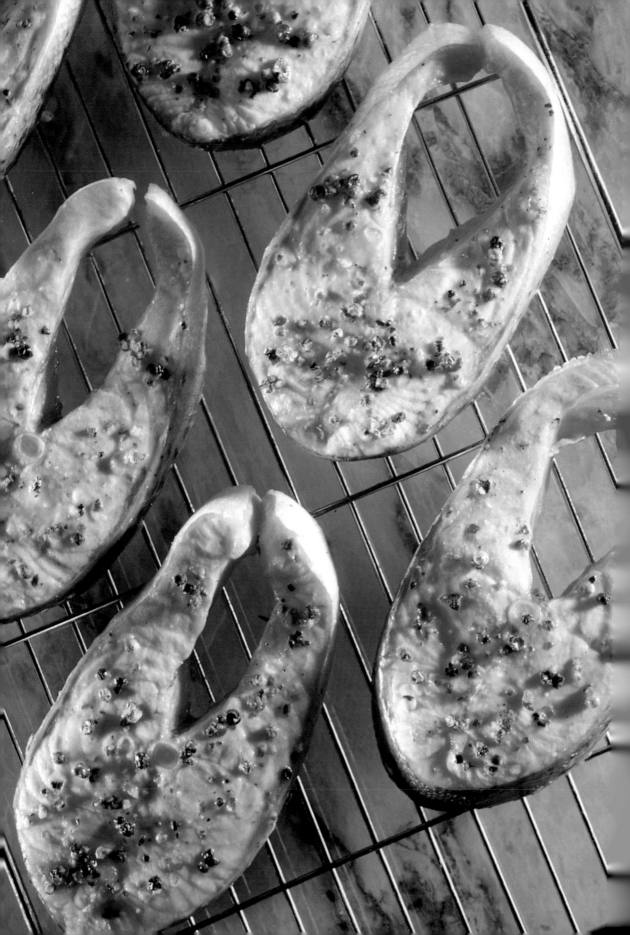

Beef, Pepper & Baby Corn Stir-Fry

This recipe is ideal for entertaining as much can be done in advance, leaving you more time with your guests. I marinate the meat in the morning and prepare the vegetables just before the guests arrive.

1 lb	lean beef filet, sliced into very thin strips	500 g
1 tbsp	cornstarch	15 mL
2 tbsp	soy sauce	25 mL
6 tbsp	dry red wine	100 mL
3 tbsp	red wine vinegar	50 mL
	Salt and freshly ground black pepper	
1 tbsp	olive or corn oil	15 mL
1	onion, finely sliced	1
2	garlic cloves, crushed	2
1	1-inch (2.5 cm) piece ginger root, grated	1
3	stalks celery, finely sliced	3
1	red bell pepper, seeded and thinly sliced	1
1	green bell pepper, seeded and thinly sliced	1
8 oz	baby corn, cut into small pieces	250 g
4 oz	brown or white mushrooms, sliced	120 g

Place the beef in a bowl. Mix together the cornstarch, soy sauce, wine and vinegar, salt and pepper in a small bowl. Pour over the meat, stir well to coat, cover and marinate in the refrigerator 2 hours or overnight.

Heat the oil in a wok or large skillet. Add the onion, garlic and ginger and stir-fry over medium heat 2 to 3 minutes. Drain the marinade from the steak and reserve, add the meat to the wok and stir-fry over high heat 3 to 4 minutes. Add the remaining vegetables and stir-fry 2 to 3 minutes.

Add the marinade and cook, stirring, until bubbly and juices thicken slightly. Adjust seasoning to taste and serve immediately with cooked noodles or brown rice. Makes 4 servings.

❖ Beef filet is expensive, but for this recipe, where it is to be cut into strips, buy the thin end piece. It should be cheaper than the thick end.

ASIAN SUPPER FOR 4

❖ Cheese and Spinach Filo Triangles (page 23)

❖ Beef, Pepper and Baby Corn Stir-Fry (opposite), served with noodles or rice

❖ Figs with Blackberry Sauce (page 146)

LEFT: *Broiled Salmon with Garlic and Peppercorns (page 39)*

PER SERVING: ¼ of recipe

Calories	310
g protein	37
g carbohydrate	14
g dietary fiber	3
g fat–total	10
g saturated fat	3
mg cholesterol	78
mg sodium	647

Beef Burgundy

A classic Burgundy dish. The flavor improves if it is made a day in advance and kept in the refrigerator. If made ahead, any fat that rises to the top and hardens can be easily removed before reheating.

2 tbsp	olive oil	25 mL
2 lb	lean round steak, cubed	1 kg
2	slices lean bacon, finely chopped	2
3	stalks celery, sliced	3
4	carrots, sliced	4
2	garlic cloves, crushed	2
1 tbsp	all-purpose flour	15 mL
2 cups	beef stock	500 mL
½ cup	dry red wine	125 mL
1	bay leaf	1
1	bouquet garni	1
	Salt and freshly ground black pepper	
12	boiling onions, peeled	12

Preheat oven to 350°F (180°C). Heat the oil in a large pan over medium heat. Add beef, a few pieces at a time; cook until browned. Drain and transfer to a large casserole dish. Add the bacon, celery, carrots and garlic to the pan and cook 2 minutes.

Stir the flour into the pan and cook 1 minute, stirring constantly. Gradually add the stock, wine, bay leaf, bouquet garni, salt and pepper. Bring to a boil and pour over the meat. Cover and bake 2 hours. Stir in the onions and bake 30 minutes or until onions and beef are tender. Remove the bouquet garni and bay leaf and adjust seasoning if necessary. Serve with boiled potatoes in their skins, fresh vegetables and crusty bread, if desired. Makes 6 or 8 servings.

PER SERVING: ⅙ of recipe

1 ▱ + 7 ▱

Calories	400
g protein	52
g carbohydrate	12
g dietary fiber	2
g fat–total	14
g saturated fat	4
mg cholesterol	129
mg sodium	279

Pork and Apricot Casserole

This recipe uses beans and dried apricots to replace some of the meat. This reduce the fat content and increases the amount of fiber. The beans and apricots also add a richness to the sauce and make the meal more filling.

1 tbsp	olive or corn oil	15 mL
1 lb	lean pork tenderloin, cubed	500 g
1	large onion, finely chopped	1
1	medium green bell pepper, seeded and sliced	1
1	medium red bell pepper, seeded and sliced	1
1	tbsp all-purpose flour	15 mL
1	15-oz (425 mL) can dried pinto beans, drained	1
1 tsp	ground turmeric	5 mL
	Salt and freshly ground black pepper	
2 cups	chicken broth	500 mL
3 oz	about ½ cup dried apricots, chopped	125 mL
1 tbsp	lemon juice	15 mL

Preheat oven to 350°F (180°C). Heat the oil in a Dutch oven or flameproof casserole dish over medium heat. Add the pork and onion and cook, stirring frequently, 5 minutes or until the pork is browned. Add the bell peppers and cook 2 minutes. Stir in the flour, beans, turmeric, salt and pepper. Gradually stir in the broth. Bring to a boil. Cover and bake 1 hour. Stir in the apricots and lemon juice. Add a little more stock if casserole is too dry. Bake 15 minutes. Serve immediately with potatoes and cooked green vegetables. Makes 4 servings.

❖ Pinto beans are an important ingredient in Mexican cooking. They have a pale pink skin and small brown blotches or speckles, which gives the name pinto, which means "painted" in Spanish.

PER SERVING: ¼ of recipe

1½ ▢ + 1½ ◨ + 6 ∅

Calories	489
g protein	47
g carbohydrate	48
g dietary fiber	12
g fat–total	12
g saturated fat	3
mg cholesterol	107
mg sodium	601

Sautéed Pork with Apple

This versatile dish can be served with potatoes and freshly cooked vegetables or with rice or pasta.

1 tbsp	all-purpose flour	15 mL
	Salt and freshly ground black pepper	
1 lb	pork tenderloin, thinly sliced crosswise, then into about 1-inch (2.5-cm) strips	500 g
2 tbsp	olive or sunflower oil	25 mL
1	medium onion, sliced	1
2	medium apples, cored and thinly sliced	2
1 tsp	dry mustard	5 mL
½ cup	chicken broth	125 mL
⅓ cup	unsweetened apple juice	75 mL

Season the flour with salt and pepper. Coat pork with flour. Heat the oil in a large nonstick skillet over medium heat. Add pork and onion and cook, turning occasionally, 4 to 5 minutes or until the pork is lightly browned. Add the apples to the pan and cook 2 to 3 minutes, stirring. Stir in the remaining ingredients and bring to a boil. Reduce heat and simmer 5 to 10 minutes or until apples are tender. Season to taste with salt and pepper and serve hot. Makes 4 servings.

PER SERVING: ¼ of recipe

1½ ▰ + 4½ ▱ + 1 ◣

Calories	364
g protein	34
g carbohydrate	17
g dietary fiber	2
g fat–total	18
g saturated fat	5
mg cholesterol	90
mg sodium	288

Lamb Rhogan

*Use less curry powder if you prefer a milder taste as this provides a
rather hot curry.*

1 tbsp	olive or sunflower oil	15 mL
1¼ lb	lean lamb cubes, fat removed	625 g
1	large onion, sliced	1
2	garlic cloves, crushed	2
1 tbsp	hot curry powder	15 mL
1 tsp	turmeric	5 mL
1 cup	chicken broth	250 mL
1	14-oz (398 mL) can chopped tomatoes	1
1	medium potato, peeled and diced	1
2	carrots, diced	2
2 tbsp	raisins	25 mL

Heat the oil in a large saucepan, add the lamb, onion and garlic
and cook, stirring occasionally, 5 minutes or until browned. Stir
in the curry powder and turmeric and cook 1 minute, stirring
constantly. Stir in the broth and tomatoes, cover and simmer 40
minutes, or until the lamb is tender. Stir in the potato, carrot
and raisins.

Cover and simmer 15 minutes or until vegetables are almost
tender. Cook, uncovered, 15 minutes or until sauce is slightly
reduced. Serve with cooked brown rice. Makes 4 servings.

❖ A good curry should not
have a watery sauce, so cook
uncovered for the last 15
minutes of cooking time until
the sauce is well reduced and
coats all the ingredients.

INDIAN MEAL FOR 4

❖ Cheese and Spinach Filo
Triangles (page 23)

❖ Lamb Rhogan (opposite)
served with rice

❖ Pears with Raspberry
Sauce (page 141)

PER SERVING: ¼ of recipe

½ ▢ + 1 ◪ + 7 ⊘ +
1 ✚✚

Calories	450
g protein	51
g carbohydrate	22
g dietary fiber	3
g fat–total	17
g saturated fat	5
mg cholesterol	153
mg sodium	471

Spicy Hungarian Goulash

Goulash is traditionally a spicy dish, but you can vary the amount and type of paprika according to your taste. My husband and I both like spicy food, so I use hot paprika.

1 tbsp	olive or sunflower oil	15 mL
2 lb	lean beef round steak, fat removed, cubes	1 kg
2	onions, thinly sliced	2
1 to 2 tbsp	hot or mild paprika	15 to 25 mL
1 tbsp	all-purpose flour	15 mL
1 tbsp	chopped fresh marjoram	15 mL
2 cups	beef stock	500 mL
	Salt and freshly ground black pepper	
3 tbsp	sour cream	50 mL

Heat the oil in a large heavy saucepan. Add the beef and onions and cook, stirring occasionally, 4 to 5 minutes or until brown. Stir in the paprika, flour and marjoram and cook, stirring, 2 minutes. Gradually stir in the stock, salt and pepper. Bring to a boil, reduce the heat, cover and simmer 1½ hours or until the beef is tender.

Spoon into warmed bowls and top with the sour cream. Sprinkle with a little paprika and serve with fresh crusty bread. Makes 4 servings.

PER SERVING: ¼ of recipe

½ 🍩 + 10 🍩

Calories	497
g protein	69
g carbohydrate	7
g dietary fiber	1
g fat–total	19
g saturated fat	7
mg cholesterol	161
mg sodium	317

Cheesy Shepherd's Pie

If you use a nonstick pan to cook the ground beef, you don't need to add any oil as it will cook in its own fat. Even with lean ground beef you can still pour off excess fat when it is cooked. This is a favorite with children.

2 lb	lean ground beef	1 kg
1	large onion, finely chopped	1
2 tbsp	tomato paste	25 mL
1	14-oz (398 mL) can tomatoes	1
1 cup	beef stock	250 mL
	Salt and freshly ground black pepper	
2 lb	potatoes, peeled and halved	1 kg
¼ cup	skim milk	60 mL
1 tbsp	soft margarine	15 mL
1 cup	frozen green peas, thawed	250 mL
¼ cup	shredded reduced-fat Cheddar cheese	60 mL

Cook the ground beef and onion in a large nonstick pan over medium heat 5 minutes, stirring to break up beef, or until browned. Drain off the excess fat. Stir in the tomato paste, tomatoes and stock. Season with salt and pepper. Bring to a boil, cover simmer 45 minutes.

Meanwhile, boil the potatoes in lightly salted water 20 to 25 minutes or until tender. Drain and mash together with the milk and margarine. Season with salt and pepper.

Preheat oven to 350°F (180°C). Stir the peas into the beef mixture. Spoon into a 1½-quart (1.5-L) casserole dish. Cover with the mashed potatoes. Bake 25 minutes or until lightly browned and bubbly. Sprinkle with the cheese. Return to oven until cheese melts. Serve hot. Makes 6 servings.

VEGETABLE THATCH PIE

❖ Replace some of the potato with carrots and parsnips for a tasty topping. Just boil them and mash them altogether.

PER SERVING: ⅙ of recipe

2 ▢ + ½ ◪ + 6½ ▨ + 1½ ▲

Calories	614
g protein	51
g carbohydrate	41
g dietary fiber	5
g fat–total	27
g saturated fat	10
mg cholesterol	151
mg sodium	431

Endive Gratin

This recipe comes from a France, where endive is very popular.

Left: Normandy Apple Flan (page 161)

❖ Belgian endive is a delicate vegetable that needs to be protected from the light to retain its white blanched color. Choose Belgian endive that is crisp, firm and white with tightly packed leaves.

8	Belgian endive heads, cleaned and trimmed	8
½ cup	chicken broth	125 mL
¼ cup	lemon juice	60 mL
1½ cups	skim milk	375 mL
4	slices cooked lean ham, halved	4
2 tbsp	soft margarine	25 mL
2 tbsp	all-purpose flour	25 mL
	Salt and freshly ground black pepper	
¾ cup	shredded Swiss cheese	175 mL

Preheat oven to 375°F (190°C). Lightly grease a casserole dish large enough to hold Belgian endive in one layer. Cook the Belgian endive in lightly salted boiling water 5 minutes. Drain and place in greased dish. Add the chicken broth and lemon juice, cover and bake 1 hour or until very tender.

Carefully remove the Belgian endive from the dish and set aside. Pour the cooking juices into a 2-cup (500-mL) measure and add enough milk to make up to 2 cups (500 mL).

When the Belgian endive is cool enough to handle, wrap a piece of ham around each head and return to the dish.

Melt the margarine in a saucepan over medium heat. Stir in the flour and cook 1 minute. Stir in the milk, bring to a boil and cook, stirring, 1 to 2 minutes or until thickened. Season with salt and pepper. Pour the sauce over the Belgian endive. Sprinkle with the cheese and bake 15 to 20 minutes or until lightly browned. Serve hot. Makes 4 servings.

PER SERVING: ¼ of recipe

½ ☐ + ½ ◆ Skim +
2 ⬤ + 1½ ▲

Calories	245
g protein	18
g carbohydrate	14
g dietary fiber	2
g fat–total	14
g saturated fat	6
mg cholesterol	39
mg sodium	699

Chicken, Spicy Sausage and Seafood Paella

There are many different versions of this popular Spanish dish. If desired, substitute the same weight of firm white fish for the mussels. Traditionally, saffron is used to color and flavor this dish. Turmeric is much cheaper but does not taste the same. Saffron is usually available in the spice section of the supermarket and you need only add a pinch in place of the turmeric for the authentic flavor.

2 tbsp	olive or corn oil	25 mL
1	large onion, finely chopped	1
2	red bell peppers, seeded and sliced	2
1	green bell pepper, seeded and sliced	1
1 lb	boneless, skinless chicken breasts, cut into 1-inch (2.5-cm) pieces	500 g
3 oz	chorizo sausage, sliced	75 g
1	8-oz (250 mL) can chopped tomatoes	1
1 cup	brown rice	250 mL
	Generous pinch of saffron or 2 tsp (10 mL) turmeric	
2 cups	chicken broth	500 mL
6 oz	peeled shrimp	175 g
6 oz	mussels in shells, scrubbed	175 g
2 tbsp	chopped fresh parsley	25 mL

Heat the oil in a large wok or paella pan over medium heat. Add the onion, garlic, bell peppers and chicken and cook, stirring occasionally, 5 minutes or until vegetables are soft. Stir in the sausage, tomatoes, rice, saffron or turmeric and broth. Bring to a boil. Reduce heat, cover and simmer 15 minutes. Stir the paella and cook, uncovered, 15 minutes.

Add the shrimp, mussels and parsley, bring back to a boil, simmer uncovered, 5 to 10 minutes or until the mussels open, the liquid is absorbed and the rice is tender. Discard any mussels that do not open. Serve immediately with crusty bread and a crisp green salad. Makes 4 to 6 servings.

FRESH MUSSELS

❖ When using fresh mussels, make sure that you discard any that remain open when tapped with your finger and any that do not open when they are cooked.

PER SERVING: ¼ of recipe

1½ ☐ + 1 ◪ + 4½ ◪

Calories	145
g protein	35
g carbohydrate	33
g dietary fiber	3
g fat–total	13
g saturated fat	3
mg cholesterol	108
mg sodium	645

Marinated Chicken and Rosemary Kebabs

This simple dish is ideal for barbecues. Serve with Greek Salad (page 48) and cooked brown rice or couscous.

1½ lb	boneless, skinless chicken breasts, trimmed and cut into 2-inch (5-cm) pieces	750 g
3 tbsp	olive oil	50 mL
3 tbsp	lemon juice	50 mL
2 tbsp	fresh rosemary leaves	25 mL
	Freshly ground black pepper	

Thread the chicken onto metal skewers and lay in a shallow dish. Mix the oil, lemon juice, rosemary and pepper together in a small bowl and pour the marinade over the kebabs. Cover and refrigerate 2 hours.

Preheat broiler. Arrange kebabs in a baking pan. Broil kebabs about 10 to 15 minutes or until the chicken is cooked through, brushing with the marinade during the first 5 minutes turning frequently. Serve hot. Makes 4 servings.

PER SERVING: ¼ of recipe

5 ⬛

Calories	272
g protein	34
g carbohydrate	0
g dietary fiber	0
g fat–total	14
g saturated fat	2
mg cholesterol	94
mg sodium	82

Spiced Chicken Brochettes with Couscous, Red Bean and Coriander Pilaf

A brochette is simply the name for a skewer on which chunks of meat are cooked. The chicken is marinated for at least 2 hours or overnight so that all the lovely flavors can develop.

4	5-oz (150 g) boneless, skinless chicken breasts	4
6 tbsp	lemon juice	90 mL
2 tbsp	olive oil	25 mL
1 tsp	paprika	5 mL
	Freshly ground black pepper	
1 tsp	ground cumin	5 mL
2 tsp	ground coriander	10 mL
8 oz	couscous	250 g
1¾ cups	cold water	425 mL
½ tsp	salt	2 mL
1	7-oz (200 mL) can red kidney beans, drained and rinsed	1
⅓ cup	raisins	75 mL
¼ cup	fresh cilantro, chopped	60 mL
	Lemon wedges to garnish	

Soak 8 wooden skewers in hot water 3 minutes to prevent burning during cooking. Slice the chicken breasts in half lengthwise and thread one strip of chicken on to each wooden skewer. Place in a shallow dish. Mix together the lemon juice, 1 tbsp (15 mL) of the olive oil, the paprika, pepper, cumin and coriander in a small bowl. Spoon over the chicken and marinate in the refrigerator 2 hours.

Place the couscous in a large bowl and stir in the 1 cup (250 mL) of the water and the salt. Let soak 5 minutes, then add remaining water and the remaining olive oil. Stir well with a fork to break up any lumps. Let stand another 10 minutes, or until the grains are slightly swollen.

❖ Pilaf, or pilau, as it is sometimes called, is usually made with rice. This variation made with couscous is a perfect foil for the Moorish flavors of the chicken brochettes.

PER SERVING: ¼ of recipe

2½ ▢ + 1½ ◪ + 5 ⊘

Calories	477
g protein	43
g carbohydrate	57
g dietary fiber	5
g fat–total	8
g saturated fat	1
mg cholesterol	83
mg sodium	653

Preheat broiler. Place chicken on a baking pan. Broil 15 to 20 minutes, turning occasionally, or until chicken is white in center. Brush with the marinade during the first 5 minutes of cooking.

Meanwhile, put the couscous in a fine metal sieve or colander and steam over boiling water 10 minutes. Stir in the kidney beans and raisins and steam another 5 minutes. Stir in half the cilantro and spoon into a serving dish. Arrange the chicken brochettes over the top of the pilaf and serve garnished with the remaining cilantro and lemon wedges. Makes 4 servings.

Georgia Chicken

The peanuts add an unexpected crunch to the sauce and make it a little bit different. Cajun seasoning is available from supermarkets in the spice section.

4	boneless, skinless chicken breasts	4
3 tbsp	soft margarine, melted	50 mL
1 tsp	Cajun seasoning	5 mL
2	medium onions, coarsely chopped	2
2 tbsp	all-purpose flour	25 mL
2 cups	skim milk	500 mL
¼ tsp	each dried thyme and oregano	1 mL
1	8-oz (250 mL) can whole-kernel corn, drained	1
¼ cup	unsalted dry-roasted peanuts	60 mL
	A pinch of cayenne pepper	

Preheat oven to 350°F (180°C). Brush the chicken with a little of the melted margarine and sprinkle with the Cajun seasoning. Place in a baking pan and bake about 30 minutes, turning halfway through cooking, or until chicken is white in center when cut with a knife.

About 15 minutes before the end of cooking time, heat the remaining margarine in a saucepan over medium heat. Add the onions and cook, stirring occasionally, until softened, 3 to 4 minutes. Stir in the flour and gradually blend in the milk. Bring to a boil, stirring constantly. Add the herbs and stir in the corn. Transfer the chicken to a serving dish, pour the sauce over the chicken and sprinkle with the peanuts and cayenne pepper. Serve hot with brown rice and cooked broccoli. Makes 4 servings.

❖ Cajun seasoning is a hot, spicy mixture redolent of the American Deep South. It is usually contains salt, so you won't need to add any more salt to the dish, but it also contains a powerful blend of herbs and spices. These may include chili powder, black pepper, garlic, allspice, coriander seed, cumin, fennel seed, cardamom, mustard, thyme, sage and oregano.

PER SERVING: ¼ of recipe

1 ▢ + ½ ◪ +
½ ◆ Skim + 4 ▨ +
½ ▲

Calories	395
g protein	36
g carbohydrate	26
g dietary fiber	3
g fat–total	17
g saturated fat	3
mg cholesterol	75
mg sodium	391

Chicken Marengo

Use a large casserole dish to enable the chicken pieces to be browned more easily. As little oil is used to brown the chicken, you may need to stir or turn the meat more frequently to prevent it sticking.

❖ Marengo means the dish is cooked in a sauce of mushrooms, tomatoes and garlic. It is said to have come from a dish that was cooked for Napoleon immediately after the battle of Marengo on June 14, 1800, from the only ingredients that were available.

1 tbsp	all-purpose flour	15 mL
	Salt and freshly ground black pepper	
4	boneless, skinless chicken breasts	4
2 tbsp	olive or sunflower oil	25 mL
1	large onion, sliced	1
2	garlic cloves, crushed	2
4 oz	button mushrooms, wiped	120 g
2	14-oz (398 mL) cans chopped tomatoes	2
½ cup	chicken broth	125 mL
2 tbsp	brandy	25 mL

Season the flour with salt and pepper. Coat the chicken breasts with the flour. Heat the oil in a large skillet or Dutch oven over medium heat. Add the chicken and cook, turning, 5 to 10 minutes or until golden brown. Remove with a slotted spoon and reserve. Add the onion, garlic and mushrooms to the skillet and cook 5 minutes, or until soft. Return the chicken to the skillet with the remaining ingredients. Season with salt and pepper. Bring to a boil. Reduce heat, cover and simmer 1 hour or until the chicken is tender.

Transfer the chicken to a warmed serving dish. If the sauce is too thin, boil briskly to reduce slightly and thicken. Spoon the sauce over the chicken and serve hot with cooked brown rice or pasta. Makes 4 servings.

PER SERVING: ¼ of recipe

1 ▮ + 4 ▮

Calories	291
g protein	30
g carbohydrate	15
g dietary fiber	3
g fat–total	11
g saturated fat	2
mg cholesterol	73
mg sodium	620

Rock Cornish Hen with Walnuts

Unlike regular chickens, Cornish hens have all dark meat.

1 tbsp	olive or sunflower oil	15 mL
4	Rock Cornish hens, thawed and rinsed	4
2	shallots, peeled and chopped	2
1 tbsp	cornstarch	15 mL
2 tbsp	cold water	25 mL
2 cups	chicken broth	500 mL
½ cup	dry white wine	125 mL
½ cup	walnut halves, toasted	125 mL
	Salt and freshly ground black pepper	
2 tbsp	chopped fresh parsley	25 mL

Preheat oven to 325°F (160°C). Heat the oil in a large Dutch oven over medium heat. Add the hens and shallots cook, turning often, until browned. Mix the cornstarch with the water and stir into the Dutch oven with the broth and wine. Stir in the walnuts, salt and pepper. Bring to a boil. Cover and bake 1½ hours or until the hens are tender. Stir in the parsley and adjust seasoning if necessary. Serve with wild rice and green vegetables. Makes 4 servings.

❖ Rock Cornish hens or Rock Cornish game hens are usually served one per person. They are available in the frozen food section in the supermarket.

PER SERVING: ¼ of recipe

½ ▰ + 12½ ▱ + 3 ◣

Calories	891
g protein	88
g carbohydrate	6
g dietary fiber	1
g fat–total	53
g saturated fat	13
mg cholesterol	268
mg sodium	1482

Catalonian Chicken

Chorizo is usually located in the meat section in major supermarkets.
If you prefer, use chicken breasts instead of chicken quarters.

SPANISH MENU

❖ Chilled Summer
Gazpacho (page 15) served
with fresh crusty bread

❖ Catalonian Chicken (opposite) served with steamed rice

❖ Spiced Apple Pie in Filo
Pastry (page 145)

1 tbsp	all-purpose flour	15 mL
	Salt and freshly ground black pepper	
4	chicken quarters, skin removed	4
2 tbsp	olive or sunflower oil	25 mL
4	shallots, peeled	4
2	garlic cloves, crushed	2
1½ cups	chicken broth	375 mL
2 tbsp	dry white wine (optional)	25 mL
2 tbsp	tomato paste	25 mL
8 oz	button mushrooms, wiped	250 g
6 oz	cooked chorizo links, sliced	175 g

Preheat oven to 350°F (180°C). Season the flour with salt and
pepper. Coat the chicken pieces with flour. Heat the oil in a Dutch
over or large flameproof casserole dish and cook the chicken until
browned all over, turning. Remove from the dish with a slotted
spoon and reserve.

Add the shallots and garlic to the Dutch oven and cook 5 minutes
or until soft. Gradually stir in the broth, wine (if using), tomato
paste. Season with salt and pepper.

Cover and bake 1 hour. Add the mushrooms and chorizo and cook
15 minutes or until the chicken is tender. Makes 4 servings.

PER SERVING: ¼ of recipe

½ ◢ + 6 ⬗ + 1 ▲
+ 1 ✚✚

Calories	431
g protein	41
g carbohydrate	8
g dietary fiber	1
g fat–total	24
g saturated fat	8
mg cholesterol	106
mg sodium	859

Rock Cornish Hens

Slow moist cooking makes the Rock Cornish hens succulent.

2 tbsp	olive or sunflower oil	25 mL
4	Rock Cornish hens, thawed and rinsed	4
2	slices lean bacon, finely chopped	2
1	onion, chopped	1
1	garlic clove, crushed	1
2	large carrots, sliced	2
1 tbsp	all-purpose flour	15 mL
1 tbsp	tomato paste	15 mL
1½ cups	chicken broth	375 mL
1 tsp	each dried thyme and rosemary	5 mL
2	bay leaves	2
	Salt and freshly ground black pepper	

Preheat oven to 325°F (160°C). Heat the oil in a large Dutch oven over medium heat. Add hens and brown on all sides. Remove with a slotted spoon and set aside.

Add the bacon, onion, garlic and carrots to the Dutch oven and cook 5 minutes or until the vegetables are soft. Stir in the flour and tomato paste and cook, stirring, 1 to 2 minutes. Gradually stir in the broth. Add the herbs, salt and pepper. Return the hens to the Dutch oven and bring the mixture to a boil.

Cover and bake 1½ hours or until hens are tender. Serve with pan juices. Makes 4 servings.

❖ Serve with boiled or mashed potatoes or Dry-Roasted Potatoes (page 168) and cooked green vegetables.

PER SERVING: ¼ of recipe

½ ◪ + 12½ ◙
+ 2½ ▲ + 1 ✚✚

Calories	856
g protein	87
g carbohydrate	9
g dietary fiber	2
g fat–total	50
g saturated fat	13
mg cholesterol	270
mg sodium	1477

Chicken Tikka

This comes from an authentic recipe from my brother's friend Mohammed. Serve with a side salad and steamed rice. If you are using wooden skewers, soak them well in water before threading on the meat to prevent them burning during cooking.

⅔ cup	low-fat plain yogurt	150 mL
1 tbsp	ground ginger	15 mL
1 tbsp	chili powder	15 mL
1 tbsp	ground coriander	15 mL
2 tsp	olive or sunflower oil	10 mL
2	garlic cloves, crushed	2
	Salt	
1 tsp	lemon juice	5 mL
4	boneless, skinless chicken breasts, cubed	4

Stir together the yogurt, spices, oil, garlic, salt and lemon juice in a large bowl. Stir in the chicken. Cover and marinate in the refrigerator overnight.

Preheat broiler. Remove chicken from marinade. Thread the chicken on to skewers and place in a baking pan. Grill 8 to 10 minutes, until cooked through, basting with the marinade during the first 5 minutes of cooking only. Makes 4 servings.

❖ Tikka is a Hindi word that roughly translated means "kebab."

❖ These skewered sticks of meat would also be ideal to cook on a grill.

PER SERVING: ¼ of recipe

½ ◆ Skim + 4 ∅

Calories	184
g protein	29
g carbohydrate	3
g dietary fiber	0
g fat–total	5
g saturated fat	1
mg cholesterol	74
mg sodium	228

Traditional Roast Chicken with Raisin and Parsley Stuffing

This dish not only tastes delicious but is surprisingly low in fat too. Use the cooking liquid from the accompanying vegetables in place of the giblet stock if desired. Removing the skin from the chicken when carving will make the meal even lower in fat.

5 lb	roasting chicken with giblets	2.5 kg
1	large onion	1
¼ cup	raisins	60 mL
2¼ cup	fresh whole-wheat bread crumbs	550 mL
6 tbsp	chopped fresh parsley	90 mL
	Salt and freshly ground black pepper	
2½ cups	water	625 mL
1 tbsp	cornstarch mixed with 2 tbsp (25 mL) cold water	15 mL

Remove the giblets and reserve. Rinse the chicken cavity with cold water and drain well. Coarsely chop half the onion and reserve remaining half for cooking with giblets. Process chopped onion, raisins, bread crumbs parsley in a food processor until the mixture binds together. Season with salt and pepper.

Preheat oven to 375°F (190°C). Lightly pack stuffing mixture into chicken cavity and truss the chicken loosely with string. Place the chicken in a roasting pan, cover with foil and roast 20 minutes per lb, plus 20 minutes extra. Remove the foil from the chicken 30 minutes before the end of cooking time. Test the chicken by inserting a skewer into the thickest part of the leg. If the juices run clear it is ready. Transfer to a serving plate. Meanwhile, rinse the giblets and place in a saucepan with the water, reserved onion and pepper. Simmer, uncovered, 1 hour.

Make the gravy: Drain the fat from the roasting pan and discard. Stir cornstarch mixture and pour into the roasting pan. Drain the giblets, reserving the stock. Pour the stock into the pan and cook, stirring occasionally over low heat until slightly thickened. Serve with the carved chicken. Makes 6 to 8 servings.

PER SERVING: ⅛ of recipe

3½ ☐ + ½ ◪ + 7 ⦸
+ 5½ ▲

Calories	915
g protein	58
g carbohydrate	58
g dietary fiber	2
g fat–total	48
g saturated fat	14
mg cholesterol	208
mg sodium	680

Cowboy's Supper

This is a quick-and-easy family supper that is convenient to make because it is cooked quickly on the stove top. Sausages and beans are a traditional combination that is popular with children. Serve with mashed potato for a campfire supper.

❖ It is much easier to persuade children to eat what is good for them if it is fun. Serve this in true western style on enamel camping plates.

1 lb	reduced-fat precooked chicken or turkey sausages	500 g
1 tbsp	olive or corn oil	15 mL
1	large onion, sliced	1
2	large carrots, diced	2
1	14-oz (398 mL) can chopped tomatoes	1
1 tbsp	dried mixed herbs	15 mL
1	8-oz (250 mL) can pork and beans	1
½ cup	vegetable or chicken stock	125 mL
	Salt and freshly ground black pepper	

Cut the sausages into bite-size pieces and set aside. Heat the oil in a large saucepan over medium heat. Add the onion and carrots and cook 5 minutes, stirring occasionally. Stir in the sausages and the remaining ingredients. Bring to a boil. Reduce heat, cover simmer 20 to 25 minutes or until the sauce has thickened slightly and the vegetables are tender. Makes 4 or 5 servings.

PER SERVING: ¼ of recipe

½ ▢ + 1 ◪ + 4 ⬨ + 2 ▲

Calories	403
g protein	29
g carbohydrate	23
g dietary fiber	6
g fat–total	23
g saturated fat	7
mg cholesterol	96
mg sodium	1308

Pasta

Pasta dishes are filling and economical, as well as a good source of carbohydrate. Try experimenting with different shapes and varieties. Some pastas are available in whole-wheat, which are higher in fiber, but any type is suitable for healthful eating, providing it is not smothered in high-fat sauces!

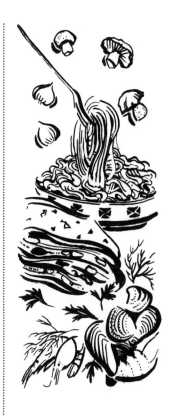

Spaghetti Tossed with Turkey and Walnuts

If you have a carbohydrate allowance per meal you can vary the amount of spaghetti to suit your needs—2 oz (60 g) of dry pasta gives approximately 35 grams of carbohydrate.

❖ Serve with a crisp green salad and finish with fresh fruit for a delicious meal in minutes.

8 oz	whole-wheat spaghetti	250 g
2 tsp	olive or sunflower oil	10 mL
10 oz	turkey ham, chopped	300 g
1	garlic clove, crushed	1
2 oz	walnuts, chopped	60 g
1	14-oz (398 mL) can chopped tomatoes	1
2 tbsp	freshly chopped parsley	25 mL
	Freshly ground black pepper	

Cook the spaghetti in boiling salted water, according to the package instructions until just tender. Drain the spaghetti and place in a serving bowl.

Meanwhile, heat the oil in a medium saucepan over medium heat. Add the turkey ham, garlic and walnuts and cook until golden, stirring constantly. Stir in the tomatoes and parsley and heat, stirring constantly 2 to 3 minutes or until piping hot. Season with black pepper. Add sauce to spaghetti and toss to combine. Serve hot. Makes 4 servings.

PER SERVING: ¼ of recipe

2½ ▢ + 1 ◩ + 3 ⊘ + 1½ ▲

Calories	445
g protein	16
g carbohydrate	55
g dietary fiber	9
g fat–total	16
g saturated fat	3
mg cholesterol	39
mg sodium	824

Seafood Lasagna

Cod is naturally low in fat and makes a refreshing change to the more traditional meat lasagna.

12 oz	cod or other white fish fillet	350 g
2½ cups	skim milk	625 mL
¼ cup	soft margarine	60 mL
¼ cup	all-purpose flour	60 mL
4 oz	peeled shrimp	120 g
2 tbsp	chopped fresh parsley	25 mL
1	7-oz (200 mL) can whole-kernel corn, drained	1
2 tsp	lemon juice	10 mL
	Salt and freshly ground black pepper	
8 to 10	green lasagna noodles, cooked	8 to 10
½ cup	shredded reduced-fat cheddar cheese	125 mL

❖ Serve with Tomato and Red Onion Salad (page 48).

Preheat oven to 350°F (180°C). Place the fish and milk in a saucepan over low heat, cover and simmer 10 to 15 minutes or until fish flakes when pierced with a fork. Reserving the cooking liquid, remove the fish and flake with a fork, removing any skin or bones.

Melt the margarine in a saucepan over low heat. Stir in the flour and cook, stirring, 1 minute. Gradually stir in the reserved cooking liquid and boil, stirring constantly, until the sauce thickens. Remove from the heat and stir in the cod, shrimp, parsley, corn and lemon juice. Season with salt and pepper.

Arrange half the noodles over the bottom of a 9-inch (23-cm)-square baking dish. Cover with half the fish mixture. Repeat the layers once more, ending with a layer of sauce.

Sprinkle the cheese over the top and bake 25 to 30 minutes or until golden brown. Makes 4 to 6 servings.

PER SERVING: ¼ of recipe

3½ ☐ + 1 ◆ Skim +
4½ ⬤ + ½ ▲

Calories	557
g protein	42
g carbohydrate	62
g dietary fiber	3
g fat–total	15
g saturated fat	3
mg cholesterol	107
mg sodium	597

Mushroom and Chicken Tagliatelle

Mushrooms are a very useful ingredient in a healthy diet. They add bulk to the dish without using meat and they are delicious and meaty in their own right. They are low in salt and carbohydrate, and have no fat, but are a good source of vegetable protein as well as important B-group vitamins and potassium.

12 oz	tagliatelle	350 g
1 tbsp	olive or corn oil	15 mL
1	small onion, finely chopped	1
1	garlic clove, crushed	1
8 oz	brown mushrooms, sliced	250 g
1	boneless, skinless chicken breast, cooked and coarsely chopped	1
2 tbsp	cornstarch	25 mL
2 tbsp	cold water	25 mL
1½ cups	chicken broth	375 mL
½ cup	2 percent low-fat milk	125 mL
	Salt and freshly ground black pepper	

Cook the tagliatelle in boiling water according to the package instructions until just tender. Drain in a colander.

Meanwhile, heat the oil in a nonstick skillet or wok over medium heat. Add the onion, garlic and mushrooms and cook 3 to 4 minutes until softened. Stir in the chicken and cook 1 to 2 minutes or until browned. Mix the cornstarch with the water and add to the pan, stirring constantly. Gradually stir in the broth and milk. Season to taste and stir until thickened. Serve spooned over the tagliatelle. Makes 4 servings.

PER SERVING: ¼ of recipe

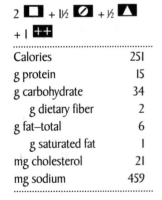

2 ☐ + 1½ ⊘ + ½ ▲
+ 1 ++

Calories	251
g protein	15
g carbohydrate	34
g dietary fiber	2
g fat–total	6
g saturated fat	1
mg cholesterol	21
mg sodium	459

Baked Zucchini, Red Pepper and Tuna Pasta

This recipe uses a fat-free white sauce, as the base for the cheese sauce, that can also be used in other recipes that require a sauce.

8 oz	pasta, preferably whole-wheat	250 g
1 tbsp	olive or sunflower oil	15 mL
1	large onion, finely chopped	1
2	medium zucchini, sliced	2
1	large red bell pepper, seeded and finely diced	1
1 tsp	dried mixed herbs	5 mL
7 oz	can tuna packed in water, drained	200 mL

Cheese Sauce

2 tbsp	cornstarch	25 mL
1½ cups	skim milk	375 mL
¾ cup	shredded reduced-fat aged Cheddar cheese	175 mL
	Salt and freshly ground black pepper	
	Freshly chopped parsley to garnish	

Preheat oven to 400°F (200°C). Lightly grease a large casserole dish. Cook the pasta in boiling water according to the package instruction until tender, drain and set aside. Meanwhile, heat the oil in a nonstick skillet over medium heat. Add the onion, zucchini and bell peppers and cook, covered, 4 to 5 minutes or until soft. Stir in the mixed herbs, tuna and pasta and mix thoroughly. Turn into greased dish.

Mix the cornstarch with a little of the milk to form a smooth paste. Heat the remaining milk in a saucepan, then pour on to the corn-starch mixture, stirring thoroughly. Return the cornstarch mixture to the saucepan, and cook, stirring constantly over low heat 1 to 2 minutes until thickened. Stir in the cheese and season with salt and pepper. Pour the cheese sauce over the pasta.

Bake 25 minutes or until golden brown. Serve sprinkled with chopped fresh parsley. Makes 4 to 6 servings.

❖ Suitable for freezing. After adding the cheese sauce, cool quickly and freeze. Thaw completely in the refrigerator and then bake as in the recipe.

PER SERVING: ¼ of recipe

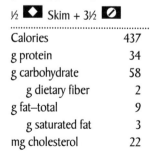

3 ▢ + 1 ◪ + ½ ◆ Skim + 3½ ⬙

Calories	437
g protein	34
g carbohydrate	58
g dietary fiber	2
g fat–total	9
g saturated fat	3
mg cholesterol	22
mg sodium	735

Ham and Tomato Pasta Sauce

For a variation, thin strips of cooked pork or chicken could be used in place of the ham.

❖ This could also be served as a delicious filling for a baked potato but if you have a carbohydrate allowance for each meal you will need to add the carbohydrate values for the potato or pasta that you serve with this sauce.

❖ 2 oz (60 g) of dry pasta gives approximately 35 g of carbohydrate or a 7-oz (200-g) potato will give approximately 40 g of carbohydrate.

2 tsp	olive or sunflower oil	10 mL
1	onion, finely chopped	1
1	garlic clove, crushed	1
1	14-oz (398 mL) can chopped tomatoes	1
1 tbsp	tomato paste	15 mL
3 tbsp	chopped fresh parsley	50 mL
4 oz	ham, cut into cubes	120 g

Heat the oil in a saucepan over medium heat. Add the onion and garlic and cook 5 minutes or until soft, stirring occasionally. Stir in the tomatoes, tomato paste and chopped parsley. Cover and simmer 5 minutes or until the sauce has thickened. Add the ham and simmer another 5 minutes. Serve over cooked whole-wheat pasta. Makes 2 servings.

PER SERVING: ½ of recipe

1 ◪ + 2 ◩ + ½ ▲ + 1 ⊞

Calories	182
g protein	14
g carbohydrate	15
g dietary fiber	3
g fat–total	8
g saturated fat	2
mg cholesterol	27
mg sodium	1200

Stir-Fried Shredded Pork and Pasta

Add some vegetables to the stir-fry if desired, such as green or red bell peppers or baby corn. Serve with a crisp green salad. I've used 8 oz (250 g) of pasta, which gives 35 g carbohydrate per serving. You can of course vary the amount of pasta, to suit your needs and appetite— 2 oz (60 g) dry weight gives approximately 35 g carbohydrate.

1 lb	lean pork, diced and trimmed of fat	500 g
4 tbsp	white wine vinegar	60 mL
2 tbsp	soy sauce	25 mL
2 tbsp	tomato paste	25 mL
8 oz	dried whole-wheat pasta	250 g
1 tbsp	olive or corn oil	15 mL
2 tsp	cornstarch	10 mL
2 tbsp	water	25 mL
1	8-oz (250 mL) can pineapple pieces in natural juice	1

Place the pork in a bowl and mix with the vinegar, soy sauce and tomato paste. Cover and marinate in the refrigerator 2 hours. Cook the pasta in boiling water according to the package instructions just until tender.

Drain the marinade mixture and reserve. Heat the oil in a nonstick skillet or wok over medium heat. Add the pork and stir-fry 4 to 5 minutes. Add the reserved marinade. Mix the cornstarch with the water and add to the pan with the pineapple pieces and juice. Bring to a boil, stirring constantly, until the sauce thickens.

Drain the pasta and return to the hot pan. Stir in the pork and sauce. Toss together and serve immediately. Makes 4 servings.

PER SERVING: ¼ of recipe

3 ☐ + 1 ◪ + 4 ∅

Calories	433
g protein	35
g carbohydrate	57
g dietary fiber	1
g fat–total	9
g saturated fat	2
mg cholesterol	60
mg sodium	497

Chicken-Sausage Sauce

Choose reduced-fat sausage and drain well after cooking to reduce the fat in the finished recipe.

2 tbsp	olive oil	25 mL
1	large onion, finely chopped	1
8 oz	boneless, skinless chicken breast, chopped	250 g
4 oz	bulk spicy pork sausages	120 g
1 cup	canned crushed tomatoes in puree	250 mL
½ cup	chicken broth	125 mL
	Salt and freshly ground black pepper	
3 tbsp	freshly chopped parsley	50 mL

Heat the oil in a nonstick skillet with lid over medium heat. Add the onion and cook 3 to 4 minutes. Add chicken and sausage and cook, stirring to break up sausage, until sausage is browned. Drain off fat.

Stir in the tomatoes and broth and bring to a boil. Cover and simmer 10 to 15 minutes, stirring occasionally. Season with salt and pepper and stir in the chopped parsley. Serve with freshly cooked pasta. Makes 4 servings.

PER SERVING: ¼ of recipe

1 � + 2½ ⊘ + 2 ▲

Calories	270
g protein	19
g carbohydrate	10
g dietary fiber	2
g fat–total	17
g saturated fat	4
mg cholesterol	55
mg sodium	875

Ten-Minute Carbonara

Friends often say they would like some recipes that can be prepared quickly when they get home from work. Well, this is ideal because it takes very little preparation. Serve with a crisp salad, and fresh crusty bread if desired.

10 oz	whole-wheat spaghetti	300 g
4 oz	mushrooms, sliced	120 g
½ cup	whipping cream	125 mL
1	egg, beaten	1
¼ cup	shredded reduced-fat cheddar cheese	60 mL
2 tbsp	chopped fresh parsley	25 mL
6 oz	lean ham, cut into thin strips	175 g
8 oz	cooked lean chicken, cut into strips	250 g
	Salt and freshly ground black pepper	

Cook the spaghetti in a large pan in boiling water just until tender. Add the mushrooms to the spaghetti 2 minutes before the end of cooking time. Beat the milk, egg, cheese and parsley together. Drain the spaghetti and return to the hot pan. Stir in the ham, chicken, milk mixture, salt and pepper. Toss together over medium heat until hot. Serve immediately. Makes 4 servings.

PER SERVING: ¼ of recipe

3 ▢ + 5 ◪ + 1 ++

Calories	495
g protein	40
g carbohydrate	56
g dietary fiber	9
g fat–total	14
g saturated fat	6
mg cholesterol	145
mg sodium	832

Red Pesto Pasta

Pesto sauce can be purchased in jars, but it is easy to make at home and you benefit from the delicious aroma and taste of fresh basil.

❖ If you don't grow your own basil, look for fresh basil leaves in the produce section of the supermarket.

½ oz	fresh basil leaves, chopped	10 g
1	garlic clove, crushed	1
1 oz	pine nuts	25 g
⅓ cup	freshly grated Parmesan cheese	75 mL
1	11-oz (300 mL) jar sun-dried tomatoes in olive oil	1
14 oz	whole-wheat pasta	400 g
4 oz	ripe olives, pitted	120 g

Place the basil, garlic, and pine nuts in a food processor or blender. Process a few seconds. Add the cheese and process a few more seconds. Add half the tomatoes, with all of the olive oil, and blend a few seconds more, to form a smooth paste.

Cook the pasta in boiling water according to the package instructions just until tender. Drain and toss with the pesto sauce, olives and remaining tomatoes. Serve immediately with a green salad. Makes 6 servings.

PER SERVING: ⅙ of recipe

1 ▢ + ½ ◩ + 1 ⊘ + 2½ ▲

Calories	268
g protein	10
g carbohydrate	27
g dietary fiber	4
g fat–total	15
g saturated fat	4
mg cholesterol	7
mg sodium	607

Yellow Split-Pea and Turkey Sauce

Using split peas means that you will need less meat for this dish. Lentils are both filling and a valuable source of soluble fiber. Remember to soak the split peas overnight before cooking.

4 oz	yellow split peas	120 g
8 oz	lean ground turkey	250 g
1	large onion, finely chopped	1
1	garlic clove, crushed	1
1½ cups	chicken broth or vegetable stock	375 mL
1	14-oz (398 mL) can chopped tomatoes	1
2 tbsp	tomato paste	25 mL
	Salt and freshly ground black pepper	

Soak the split peas overnight in plenty of cold water. Rinse thoroughly and place in a saucepan with fresh water over medium heat. Boil rapidly 10 minutes. Rinse and drain. Place the turkey, onion and garlic in a nonstick pan over medium heat and cook 3 to 4 minutes, stirring to break up turkey. Add the drained split peas and cook 1 to 2 minutes, stirring occasionally. Add the remaining ingredients and mix well. Bring to a boil. Reduce heat, cover and simmer, stirring occasionally, 30 to 40 minutes, or until peas are tender. Serve with freshly cooked pasta and a crisp salad. Makes 4 servings.

PER SERVING: ¼ of recipe

1 ▢ + 1 ◪ + 2½ ◙ + 1 ✚✚

Calories	247
g protein	22
g carbohydrate	27
g dietary fiber	4
g fat–total	7
g saturated fat	2
mg cholesterol	41
mg sodium	699

Breads

Although breads are high in carbohydrate, they can be an important part of a meal plan, particularly breads that are high in fiber. This collection of recipes includes favorite quick breads made with fruit and whole-grain yeast breads. Most breads freeze well. Cool after baking, slice, wrap well and freeze up to three months.

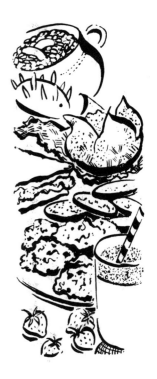

Baking-Powder Biscuits

Serve these hot for breakfast or as an accompaniment to a light lunch or supper.

2 cups	all-purpose flour	500 mL
4 tsp	baking powder	20 mL
½ tsp	salt	2 mL
2½ tbsp	soft margarine	40 mL
¾ cup	skim milk	175 mL

Preheat oven to 450°F (235°C). Combine flour, baking powder and salt in a medium bowl. Cut in margarine until mixture resembles coarse cornmeal. Stir in milk to make a soft dough. Turn out dough on a lightly floured board. Knead lightly and roll out to ½-inch (1-cm) thickness. Cut into rounds with a 1½-inch (3.5-cm) cutter. Arrange on a baking sheet. Bake 10 to 12 minutes or until puffed and golden brown. Makes 24 (1½-inch/3.5-cm) biscuits.

PER SERVING: ½ of recipe

☐ + ½ ▲ + ++	
Calories	52
g protein	1
g carbohydrate	9
g dietary fiber	0
g fat–total	1
g saturated fat	0
mg cholesterol	0
mg sodium	120

Buttermilk Cornbread

1 cup	cornmeal	250 mL
½ cup	all-purpose flour	125 mL
½ tsp	baking soda	2 mL
1 tsp	baking powder	5 mL
1 tsp	sugar	5 mL
2 tbsp	canola oil	25 mL
1	egg lightly beaten	1
1 cup	buttermilk	250 mL

Preheat oven to 450°F (235°C). Grease an 8-inch (20-cm)-square baking pan. Combine, cornmeal, flour, soda, baking powder and sugar in a medium bowl. Combine oil, egg and buttermilk in another bowl. Add to cornmeal mixture and stir just until moistened. Pour into prepared pan. Bake 20 to 25 minutes or until golden brown. Cut into 8 rectangles. Makes 8 pieces.

PER SERVING: ⅛ of recipe

1½ ☐ + 1 ▲

Calories	146
g protein	4
g carbohydrate	22
g dietary fiber	2
g fat–total	5
g saturated fat	1
mg cholesterol	28
mg sodium	165

Banana Bread

The dates add bulk to the mixture and replace the sugar and fat usually required in a cake recipe. Why not try replacing the sugar in some of your own recipes with a date puree? Dates contain around half the carbohydrate and calories as the same weight of sugar.

❖ Best eaten within two days. Suitable for freezing.

❖ An excellent way to use up bananas when they have started to get too soft to enjoy raw.

6 oz	pitted dried dates	175 g
½ cup	water	125 mL
1	egg	1
1 cup	mashed ripe bananas (about 2 large)	250 mL
1¾ cups	all-purpose flour	425 mL
1 tsp	baking powder	5 mL
¼ tsp	salt	1 mL
¼ tsp	baking soda	1 mL
1 tsp	ground cinnamon	5 mL
¼ cup	chopped walnuts	60 mL

Preheat oven to 350°F (180°C). Grease a 9 x 5 inch (23 x 13 cm) loaf pan and line with waxed paper. Place the dates and water in a saucepan and simmer about 5 minutes or until the dates are soft. Mash with a fork until the dates are pureed. Allow to cool slightly. Beat in the egg and bananas. Mix together the flour, baking powder, salt, soda and cinnamon in a medium bowl. Stir the date mixture into the flour mixture just until flour is moistened. Stir in the walnuts.

Spoon the mixture into the prepared pan and smooth the surface. Bake 1 hour or until a skewer inserted in the center comes out clean. Cover with foil if becoming too brown. Allow to cool in the pan 15 minutes before turning out on a wire rack to cool completely. Cut into 14 slices. Makes 1 loaf.

PER SERVING: ¼ of recipe

I ▢ + I ▰ + ½ ◣

Calories	124
g protein	3
g carbohydrate	25
g dietary fiber	2
g fat–total	2
g saturated fat	0
mg cholesterol	15
mg sodium	92

Raisin-Nut Muffins

Muffins are usually very high in calories. However, by cutting down on the sugar and fat content and increasing the fiber by using whole-wheat flour, these muffins are both nutritious and tasty to eat.

1⅓ cups	whole-wheat flour	325 mL
1 cup	all-purpose flour	250 mL
½ tsp	salt	2 mL
2 tbsp	baking powder	25 mL
2 tbsp	sugar	25 mL
¼ cup	soft margarine, melted	60 mL
2	eggs, lightly beaten	2
1¼ cup	skim milk	300 mL
2 tsp	vanilla extract	10 mL
½ cup	raisins	125 mL
¼ cup	slivered almonds	60 mL

Preheat oven to 400°F (200°C). Line a muffin pan with 12 paper cups. Sift the flours, salt and baking powder into a large bowl, adding any bran remaining in the sifter back into the bowl. In another bowl, mix together the sugar, melted margarine, eggs, milk and vanilla. Stir into the flour mixture just until flour is moistened. Stir in raisins and almonds.

Spoon the mixture evenly into the paper cups, filling about ⅔ full. Bake 25 minutes or until golden. Serve warm or cool slightly before serving. Makes 12 muffins.

❖ Muffins can make a delicious treat for a lazy weekend breakfast. Serve with fresh fruit for a substantial start to the day with tea or coffee and the newspapers.

PER SERVING: ½ of recipe

1½ ☐ + ½ ◪ + ½ ⬚ + 1 ◣

Calories	186
g protein	6
g carbohydrate	28
g dietary fiber	2
g fat–total	7
g saturated fat	1
mg cholesterol	36
mg sodium	331

Apricot-Pecan Loaf

This could also be served as a dessert.

❖ Best eaten within 1 to 2 days. Suitable for freezing.

1⅓ cups	whole-wheat flour	325 mL
1⅓ cups	all-purpose flour	325 mL
1 tbsp	baking powder	15 mL
2 tsp	cinnamon	10 mL
½ cup	sugar	125 mL
½ cup	soft margarine, melted	125 mL
2	eggs, lightly beaten	2
½ cup	skim milk	125 mL
1	14-oz (398 mL) can apricots in juice, drained and chopped	1
½ cup	pecan nuts, chopped	125 mL
	Grated peel of 1 orange	

Preheat oven to 350°F (180°C). Lightly grease an 11 x 7 inch (28 x 18 cm) baking pan and line bottom with waxed paper. Sift together the flours, baking powder and cinnamon into a large bowl, adding any bran remaining in the sifter back into the bowl. Stir in the sugar. Add the melted margarine, eggs and milk and stir until flour is moistened. Fold in the chopped apricots, nuts and grated orange peel. Pour into prepared pan. Bake 40 minutes or until golden and a skewer inserted in center comes out clean. Cool in the pan and cut into 16 slices. Makes 1 loaf.

PER SERVING: 1/16 of recipe

1 ▢ + ½ ◩ + ½ ✳ + 2 ▲

Calories	196
g protein	4
g carbohydrate	26
g dietary fiber	2
g fat–total	9
g saturated fat	1
mg cholesterol	27
mg sodium	134

Lemon-Sesame Bread

The lemon peel and juice add a lemony flavor to this bread accented with sesame seeds. It is best eaten within 2 to 3 days.

½ cup	soft margarine	125 mL
¼ cup	sugar	60 mL
2	eggs lightly beaten	2
1¼ cups	all-purpose flour	300 mL
½ cup	whole-wheat flour	125 mL
1 tsp	baking powder	5 mL
1 tsp	baking soda	5 mL
⅔ cup	nonfat plain yogurt	150 mL
2 tbsp	sesame seeds	25 mL
	Grated peel and juice of large lemon	

Preheat oven to 325°F (160°C). Grease a 9 x 5 inch (23 x 13 cm) loaf pan and line with waxed paper. Cream the margarine and sugar together, then gradually beat in the eggs. Sift the flours, baking powder and soda into a large bowl, adding any bran remaining in the sifter back into the bowl. Stir flour mixture and yogurt alternately into egg mixture. Stir in the sesame seeds, grated lemon peel and juice. Spoon into prepared pan and smooth the surface.

Bake about 1 hour or until golden and a skewer inserted in the center comes out clean. Cool on a wire rack. Cut into 14 slices. Makes 1 loaf.

❖ Store in an airtight pan. Suitable for freezing.

❖ These days, everyone should be trying to eat a low-fat, high-fiber diet, so don't keep these recipes to yourself!

PER SERVING: ¼ of recipe

1 ▢ + 1½ ▲

Calories	152
g protein	4
g carbohydrate	16
g dietary fiber	1
g fat–total	8
g saturated fat	1
mg cholesterol	31
mg sodium	195

Farmhouse Fruit Scones

You may need to use all of the egg and milk if the mixture seems dry as this will vary with the flour used. Use a little extra milk for brushing the tops of the scones before baking.

❖ They are best eaten the same day or may be frozen.

1¼ cups	all-purpose flour	300 mL
½ cup	whole-wheat flour	125 mL
2½ tsp	baking powder	12 mL
½ tsp	salt	2 mL
3 tbsp	soft margarine	50 mL
¼ cup	sugar	60 mL
½ cup	raisins	125 mL
1	egg beaten with enough skim milk to make ½ cup	125 mL
	Milk for brushing	

Preheat oven to 425°F (220°C). Sift the flours, baking powder and salt into a large bowl, adding any bran remaining in the sifter back into the bowl. Cut in the margarine until the mixture resembles bread crumbs. Stir in the sugar and raisins. Gradually add enough of the egg and milk mixture to form a soft dough.

Knead the mixture on a lightly floured surface and roll out to about ½-inch (1-cm) thickness. Cut into 2-inch (5-cm) rounds, rerolling the trimmings. Place on a floured baking sheet and brush the tops with a little milk. Bake 10 to 12 minutes or until puffed and golden. Serve warm or cool on a wire rack. Makes about 14 scones.

PER SERVING: ¹⁄₁₄ of recipe

1 ☐ + ½ ◢ + ½ ▲

Calories	116
g protein	3
g carbohydrate	20
g dietary fiber	1
g fat–total	3
g saturated fat	1
mg cholesterol	15
mg sodium	171

Ginger and Date Bread

Dried dates are naturally sweet and therefore no extra sugar is added to this bread. Pureed dates can be used to replace some or all of the sugar in some cakes, but remember to add their carbohydrate value when calculating your own recipes.

❖ This bread is best eaten within 1 to 2 days, or it may be frozen.

½ cup	skim milk	125 mL
5 oz	pitted dried dates, coarsely chopped	150 g
1¼ cups	all-purpose flour	300 mL
½ cup	whole-wheat flour	125 mL
2 tsp	baking powder	10 mL
1 tsp	baking soda	5 mL
2 tsp	ground ginger	10 mL
1 tsp	ground cinnamon	5 mL
½ cup	soft margarine	125 mL
1 oz	ground almonds	25 g
3	eggs, beaten	3
2 tbsp	water	25 mL

Preheat oven to 350°F (180°C). Grease a 9 x 5 inch (23 x 13 cm) loaf pan and line with waxed paper. Place the milk and dates in a saucepan and cook over low heat 5 minutes or until the dates are soft. Set aside.

Sift together the flour, baking powder, soda and spices into a large bowl, adding any bran remaining in the sifter back into the bowl. Cut in the margarine until the mixture resembles fine bread crumbs. Stir in the ground almonds. Gradually beat in the beaten eggs and finally stir in the water and date mixture. Beat well to combine. Spoon the mixture into prepared pan and smooth the surface.

Bake 35 to 40 minutes or until the bread is browned and a skewer inserted into the center comes out clean. Cool on a wire rack. Cut into 14 slices. Makes 1 loaf.

PER SERVING: ¼ of recipe

1 ▢ + ½ ▱ + 1½ ▲

Calories	165
g protein	4
g carbohydrate	20
g dietary fiber	2
g fat–total	8
g saturated fat	2
mg cholesterol	46
mg sodium	215

Apricot and Raisin Bread

A moist fruit loaf which is high in fiber and low in fat.

❖ Wrap well and store in an airtight container. It will keep 3 to 4 days, or alternatively it can be frozen.

1 cup	All-bran cereal	250 mL
4 oz	dried ready-to-eat apricots, chopped	120 g
¾ cup	raisins	175 mL
1 cup	strong hot tea	250 mL
¾ cup	all-purpose flour	175 mL
2 tsp	baking powder	10 mL
2	eggs beaten	2

Preheat oven to 350°F (180°C). Grease a 9 x 5 inch (23 x 13 cm) loaf pan and line with waxed paper. Place the cereal, apricots, raisins and tea in a bowl and mix well. Let stand 15 to 20 minutes. Stir in the flour, baking powder and eggs and mix well. Spoon into prepared pan and smooth the surface.

Bake 45 to 50 minutes or until a skewer inserted in the center comes out clean. Cool on a wire rack. Cut into 14 slices. Makes 1 loaf.

PER SERVING: ¹⁄₁₄ of recipe

1 ▢ + ½ ◪

Calories	96
g protein	3
g carbohydrate	22
g dietary fiber	3
g fat–total	1
g saturated fat	0
mg cholesterol	30
mg sodium	132

Cherry and Walnut Bread

When making quick breads in which the fat and sugar are creamed together, you can usually reduce the amount of sugar by half as I have in this recipe.

½ cup	soft margarine	125 mL
¼ cup	sugar	60 mL
1	egg, lightly beaten	1
2 cups	all-purpose flour	500 mL
1 tbsp	baking powder	15 mL
1 tsp	apple pie spice	5 mL
	Pinch of salt	
½ cup	chopped walnuts	125 mL
4 oz	glacé cherries, rinsed, dried and chopped	120 g
¾ cup	skim milk	175 mL

Preheat oven to 350°F (180°C). Grease a 9 x 5 inch (23 x 13 cm) loaf pan and line with waxed paper. Beat the margarine and sugar together until pale and creamy. Gradually beat in the egg. Sift the flour, baking powder, spice and salt together into a large bowl. Stir in the walnuts and cherries. Stir the flour mixture and milk alternately into the creamed mixture to make a smooth batter. Pour the mixture into prepared pan.

Bake 1¼ hours or until a skewer inserted in the center comes out clean. Cool in the pan 10 minutes before turning out on to a wire rack to cool completely. Cut into 12 to 14 slices. Makes 1 loaf.

❖ Best eaten within 2 to 3 days. Suitable for freezing. Store in an airtight container.

PER SERVING: 1/12 of recipe

3 + 1½ + 2

Calories	234
g protein	4
g carbohydrate	30
g dietary fiber	1
g fat–total	11
g saturated fat	2
mg cholesterol	18
mg sodium	197

Cheese and Bacon Bread

A savory bread that is delicious served warm.

1¼ cups	all-purpose flour	300 mL
¾ cup	whole-wheat flour	175 mL
1 tsp	baking soda	5 mL
½ tsp	cream of tartar	2 mL
½ tsp	dried mustard powder	2 mL
½ cup	soft margarine	125 mL
4 oz	Canadian bacon, finely chopped	120 g
1 cup	shredded reduced-fat Cheddar cheese	250 mL
5	green onions, finely chopped	5
1	egg, lightly beaten	1
½ cup	skim milk	125 mL

Preheat oven to 400°F (200°C). Grease a 9 x 5 inch (23 x 13 cm) loaf pan and line with waxed paper. Sift the flours, soda, cream of tartar, and mustard powder into a bowl, adding any bran remaining in the sifter back into the bowl. Cut in the margarine until the mixture resembles bread crumbs. Stir in the bacon, 3/4 of the cheese and the green onions. Beat the egg and milk together and stir into the flour mixture until moistened. Spoon into prepared pan and smooth the top. Sprinkle with remaining cheese.

Bake 35 to 40 minutes or until a skewer inserted in the center comes out clean. Allow to cool in the pan 5 minutes, before turning out on to a wire rack. Cut into about 12 slices. Serve warm or cold. Makes 1 loaf.

PER SERVING: ½ of recipe

1 ▢ + ½ ⊘ + 2½ ▲

Calories	228
g protein	7
g carbohydrate	17
g dietary fiber	1
g fat–total	15
g saturated fat	5
mg cholesterol	30
mg sodium	320

Whole-Wheat Bread

Easy-blend dried yeast should be stirred into the dry ingredients before adding the water, unlike fresh or traditional dried yeast that needs to be added to liquid first.

❖ Best eaten the same day. Suitable for freezing.

2 cups	bread flour	500 mL
1½ cups	whole-wheat flour	375 mL
1 tbsp	sugar	15 mL
2 tsp	salt	10 mL
1	package active dried yeast	1
¼ cup	soft margarine	60 mL
1¼ cups	skim milk, heated to 125°F (50°C)	300 mL

Place the flours, sugar, salt and yeast in a large bowl. Cut in the margarine and add enough milk to make a soft dough. Turn out on a lightly floured board and knead 10 to 15 minutes until smooth and elastic.

Place in an oiled bowl, cover and let rise in a warm place until doubled in size, about 1 hour. Punch down dough. Let rest 10 minutes. Grease a 9 x 5 inch (23 x 13 cm) loaf pan. Shape dough into a loaf and place in prepared pan. Let rise in a warm place until the dough is almost to the top of the pan, about 45 minutes. Preheat oven to 350°F (180°C).

Bake 50 minutes or until browned. Cool on a wire rack. Cut into about 20 slices. Makes 1 loaf.

PER SERVING: ½₀ of recipe

1 ☐ + ½ ▲

Calories	108
g protein	4
g carbohydrate	18
g dietary fiber	1
g fat–total	3
g saturated fat	1
mg cholesterol	0
mg sodium	257

Granary Loaf

Homemade bread is delicious served warm. I find it easier to make using a table-top electric mixer with a dough hook.

❖ Best eaten the same day. Suitable for freezing.

2 cups	bread flour	500 mL
1 cup	whole-wheat flour	250 mL
½ cup	rye flour	125 mL
1 tbsp	sugar	15 mL
2 tsp	salt	10 mL
1	package active dried yeast	1
3 tbsp	sunflower oil or corn oil	50 mL
1¼ cups	water, heated to 125°F (50°C)	300 mL

Place the flours, sugar, salt and yeast in a large bowl. Stir in the oil and enough water to make a soft dough. Turn out on a lightly floured board and knead 10 to 15 minutes until smooth and elastic.

Place in an oiled bowl, cover and let rise in a warm place until doubled in size, about 1 hour. Punch down dough. Let rest 10 minutes. Grease a 9 x 5 inch (23 x 13 cm) loaf pan. Shape dough into a loaf and place in prepared pan. Let rise in a warm place until the dough is almost to the top of the pan, about 45 minutes. Preheat oven to 350°F (180°C).

Bake 50 minutes or until browned. Cool on a wire rack. Cut into about 20 slices. Makes 1 loaf.

PER SERVING: ⅟₂₀ of recipe

1 ▢ + ½ ▲

Calories	102
g protein	3
g carbohydrate	17
g dietary fiber	1
g fat–total	3
g saturated fat	0
mg cholesterol	0
mg sodium	222

Hot Cross Buns

To make the buns in advance, allow to cool unglazed before freezing.
Heat thawed buns in a hot oven 2 to 3 minutes to warm, then glaze
as in the recipe before serving.

❖ Best eaten the same day.
Suitable for freezing.

2¾ cups	bread flour	675 mL
1 cup	whole-wheat flour	250 mL
1 tsp	salt	5 mL
1 tsp	apple pie spice	5 mL
½ tsp	ground cinnamon	2 mL
½ cup	soft margarine	125 mL
1	package active dried yeast	1
¼ cup	sugar	60 mL
1 cup	dried currants	250 mL
½ cup	skim milk, heated to 125°F (50°F)	125 mL
1	egg, beaten	1
¼ cup	warm water	60 mL

Glaze		
1 tbsp	reduced-sugar apricot jam	15 mL
3 tbsp	water	50 mL

Sift the flours, salt and spices into a large bowl, adding any bran
remaining in the sifter back to the bowl. Cut in the margarine. Stir
in the yeast, sugar and currants. Make a well in the center and add
the milk, egg and enough water to form a soft dough. Turn dough
out on a lightly floured surface and knead until smooth and elastic.
Place in an oiled bowl, cover with plastic wrap and let rise in a
warm place until doubled in size, 1 to 1½ hours.

Punch down the dough and shape into 14 balls. Let rest 10
minutes. Grease 2 baking sheets. Place well apart on sheets and
flatten slightly. Cover with plastic wrap and let rise 30 minutes.

Preheat oven to 400°F (180°C). Remove the plastic wrap and slash
a cross in each bun. Bake 15 to 20 minutes. Heat the jam and
water together over low heat and use to brush over the buns while
still hot. Cool on a wire rack. Makes 14 rolls.

PER SERVING: ¼ of recipe

1½ ☐ + ½ ◪ + ½ ✳

+ 1½ ▲

Calories	222
g protein	5
g carbohydrate	35
g dietary fiber	2
g fat–total	8
g saturated fat	1
mg cholesterol	15
mg sodium	225

Cakes and Cookies

Many people are concerned that they will be unable to eat cakes and cookies once they have been diagnosed with diabetes. It is still possible to eat them occasionally as part of an overall healthful diet. The recipes in this section have been developed using as little sugar as possible, together with high-fiber ingredients such as whole-wheat flour or oats as the main ingredients. Some recipes have no added sugar but rely upon the natural sweetness of dried fruit. Because of the reduced sugar and fat content, the cakes and cookies are best eaten within a few days or they may be frozen in convenient portions and used as required. This ensures that they are eaten at their best.

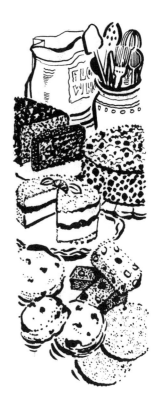

Carrot and Banana Cake

A pretty two-layer cake that can also be made in a 13 x 9 inch (33 x 23 cm) pan and cut into 24 squares—ideal to take on a picnic.

❖ Best eaten within 2 days. Suitable for freezing.

2 cups	all-purpose flour	500 mL
1 tbsp	baking powder	15 mL
1½ tsp	baking soda	7 mL
1½ tsp	pumpkin pie spice mix	7 mL
¼ cup	packed light brown sugar	60 mL
3	eggs, separated	3
1	small ripe banana, mashed	1
1	large carrot, peeled, grated ½ cup	125 mL
⅓ cup	vegetable oil	75 mL
½ cup	buttermilk	125 mL
1 tsp	vanilla extract	5 mL
1 tsp	banana extract	5 mL
2	small bananas, sliced	2
1 cup	frozen whipped nondairy dessert topping	250 mL
	Dash nutmeg	

Preheat oven to 350°F (180°C). Lightly grease two 8-inch (20-cm) baking pans. Stir together flour, baking powder, baking soda, spice mix and sugar in a bowl. Combine egg yolks, banana, carrot, oil and buttermilk. Stir into dry ingredients and beat well.

Whip eggs whites and fold into mixture. Pour into prepared pans. Bake 30 to 35 minutes or until a skewer inserted into the center comes out clean. Allow to cool in the pan a few minutes, then turn out on to a wire rack to cool completely. Place one half sliced bananas on one layer, top with one half frozen whipped topping. Place second layer on top, use remaining banana slices and topping. Sprinkle with a dash of nutmeg, if desired. Makes 24 squares. If using a 13 x 9 inch (33 x 23 cm) pan, cut into 24 squares.

PER SERVING: ⅟₂₄ of recipe

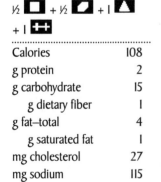

½ ▢ + ½ ◪ + 1 ◭
+ 1 ▥

Calories	108
g protein	2
g carbohydrate	15
g dietary fiber	1
g fat–total	4
g saturated fat	1
mg cholesterol	27
mg sodium	115

Chocolate and Strawberry Roll

Our family is used to a low-sugar diet. My mother has cooked this way since my grandfather developed diabetes. When I served this dessert to a colleague of my husband, we had to laugh when he added extra sugar to a low-sugar dessert!

3	eggs	3
½ cup plus 1 tsp	sugar	130 mL
½ cup	all-purpose flour	125 mL
½ cup	whole-wheat flour	125 mL
2 tbsp	unsweetened cocoa powder	25 mL
1 tbsp	warm water	15 mL

Filling

1	8-oz (250 g) package light cream cheese, softened	1
2 to 3 tbsp	granulated artificial sweetener (or to taste)	25 to 50 mL
8 oz	fresh strawberries, hulled and sliced	250 g

Preheat oven to 425°F (220°C). Grease a 13 x 9 inch (33 x 23 cm) baking pan. Using an electric mixer, beat the eggs and the ½ cup (125 mL) sugar together 5 minutes or until pale and thick and the beaters leaves a trail in the mixture for a few seconds when lifted.

Sift the flours and cocoa together. Fold carefully with the water into the egg mixture. Pour the mixture into prepared pan, tapping into the corners to cover the surface evenly. Bake 8 to 10 minutes or until cake springs back when lightly touched with a finger tip.

Sprinkle a sheet of waxed paper with 1 tsp (5 mL) sugar. Turn out cake on waxed paper and remove the lining paper. Trim cake edges very thinly and roll up with the clean paper inside. Cool completely on a wire rack. Beat the cream cheese and sweetener together until light and fluffy. Unroll the cake carefully and spread with cheese mixture. Scatter the strawberries over cheese and roll up carefully. Cut into slices. Makes 10 to 12 servings.

PER SERVING: *1/10* of recipe

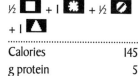

Calories	145
g protein	5
g carbohydrate	19
g dietary fiber	2
g fat–total	6
g saturated fat	3
mg cholesterol	67
mg sodium	159

Spiced Mandarin Gâteau

This elegant dessert is perfect for entertaining. I use all-purpose flour for the cake as I find it gives a better result than whole-wheat flour. If you prefer, you could use half whole-wheat and half all-purpose.

4	eggs	4
½ cup plus 2 tsp	sugar	135 mL
1 cup	all-purpose flour	250 mL
¼ tsp	ground ginger	1 mL
¼ tsp	ground cinnamon	1 mL
¼ cup	margarine, melted and cooled	60 mL

Filling

1 cup	whipping cream	250 mL
2 tbsp	granulated artificial sweetener	25 mL
1	11-oz (300 mL) can mandarin segments in natural juice, drained	1

Preheat oven to 375°F (190°C). Grease a 13 x 9 inch (33 x 23 cm) baking pan. Using an electric mixer, beat the eggs and the ½ cup (125 mL) sugar together 5 minutes or until pale and thick and the beaters leave a trail in the mixture for a few seconds when lifted.

Sift the flour and spices together. Fold carefully into the egg mixture. Finally, fold in the margarine. Pour the mixture into prepared pan. Bake 15 to 20 minutes or until cake springs back when lightly touched with a finger tip. Sprinkle a sheet of waxed paper with the 2 tsp (10 mL) sugar. Turn out cake on the waxed paper and remove the lining paper. Trim cake edges very thinly and roll up with the clean paper inside. Cool completely on a wire rack.

Whip the cream cheese and sweetener together until stiff. Unroll the cake carefully and spread with ¾ of the cream. Reserve 8 mandarin segments for decoration, arrange remaining segments over the cream, reroll the sponge carefully, sprinkle with a little sweetener (optional) and place on a serving dish. Pipe the reserved cream down the center of the roll and decorate with the remaining mandarin segments. Refrigerate until ready to serve. Makes 10 to 12 servings.

PER SERVING: ⅟₁₀ of recipe

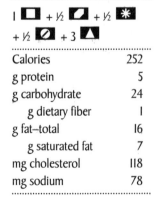

Calories	252
g protein	5
g carbohydrate	24
g dietary fiber	1
g fat–total	16
g saturated fat	7
mg cholesterol	118
mg sodium	78

Pinolata

This is an Italian dessert cake, which can be served with a fresh fruit salad.

2	eggs	2
¼ cup	sugar	60 mL
	Grated peel of 1 lemon	
¾ cup	soft margarine	175 mL
2¼ cups	all-purpose flour	550 mL
½ cup	dry sherry	125 mL
1 tsp	vanilla extract	5 mL
2 oz	pine nuts	60 g

Preheat oven to 350°F (180°C). Grease a deep 9-inch (23-cm) cake pan and line bottom with waxed paper. Whisk the eggs and sugar together until pale and creamy. Beat in the lemon peel, margarine, flour, sherry and vanilla. Mix until well blended and smooth. Pour into prepared pan. Sprinkle the pine nuts over the top. Bake 30 minutes or until a skewer inserted into the center comes out clean. Serve warm. Makes 12 servings.

PINE NUTS

❖ Pine nuts are a luxury item. They are quite expensive. The high cost is attributed to the difficulty in separating them from the pine cone in which they grow. Buy pine nuts in small quantities and use them up quickly. They go rancid rapidly because of their high fat content. Store unused portion in the freezer.

PER SERVING: ½ of recipe

1½ ▢ + 3 ◤

Calories	247
g protein	5
g carbohydrate	23
g dietary fiber	1
g fat–total	15
g saturated fat	3
mg cholesterol	35
mg sodium	117

Apricot Upside-Down Cake

A variation on the traditional pineapple upside-down cake. The sugar content has been reduced in this recipe by using fruit canned in juice rather than syrup. I have also halved the amount of sugar in the sponge recipe compared with a traditional mixture.

❖ You can vary the fruit in an upside-down cake to suit whatever is at hand. Peach slices or halves are a good choice. Try pear halves or pitted cherries; they are especially delicious when a little cocoa powder is added to the cake batter.

1	14-oz (398 mL) can apricot halves in natural juice	1
2 tbsp	granulated artificial sweetener	25 mL
¼ cup	soft margarine	60 mL
⅓ cup	sugar	75 mL
1	egg	1
1¾ cups	cake flour, sifted	425 mL
1 tsp	baking powder	5 mL
½ tsp	vanilla extract	2 mL
¼ cup	skim milk	60 mL

Preheat oven to 350°F (180°C). Grease a 9-inch (23-cm) cake pan and line with waxed paper. Drain the apricot halves, reserving the juice. Arrange the apricots flat side down in the bottom of prepared pan. Mix ¼ of the apricot juice with the sweetener and spoon over the apricots.

Beat margarine and sugar together until creamy. Beat in eggs, one at a time. Sift together flour and baking powder. Beat into creamed mixture alternately with milk.

Spoon the batter over the apricots. Bake in the center of the oven about 35 minutes or until golden and firm to the touch. Turn out on a serving plate and remove the lining paper. Serve warm. Makes 10 servings.

PER SERVING: ⅒ of recipe

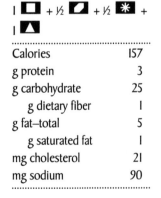

Calories	157
g protein	3
g carbohydrate	25
g dietary fiber	1
g fat–total	5
g saturated fat	1
mg cholesterol	21
mg sodium	90

Coconut and Cherry Fingers

These will keep for up to two days in an airtight tin or they may be frozen for longer storage.

1¾ cups	all-purpose flour	425 mL
2 tsp	baking powder	10 mL
½ cup	soft margarine	125 mL
⅓ cup	sugar	75 mL
⅔ cup	shredded coconut	150 mL
4 oz	glacé cherries, washed, dried and chopped	120 g
1	egg, lightly beaten	1
2 tbsp	lemon juice	25 mL
¾ cup	skim milk	175 mL

Preheat oven to 325°F (160°C). Grease an 11 x 7 inch (28 x 18 cm) baking pan and line bottom with waxed paper. Mix the flour and baking powder together in a large bowl. Cut in the margarine until the mixture resembles bread crumbs. Stir in the sugar, coconut and cherries. Stir in the egg and lemon juice and enough milk to make a soft batter. Spoon prepared pan. Bake 40 to 45 minutes or until golden brown and firm. Turn out on to a wire rack. When cooled, cut into fingers. Makes 16.

❖ Suitable for freezing. I cut cakes into slices before freezing so that individual pieces may be taken out when required. These fingers are ideal to include in lunch boxes as a snack.

PER SERVING: ⅟₁₆ of recipe

I ▢ + ½ ✳ + 1½ ▲ + I ➕

Calories	167
g protein	2
g carbohydrate	23
g dietary fiber	1
g fat–total	8
g saturated fat	2
mg cholesterol	13
mg sodium	118

Chocolate Squares

Decorate these squares could with a little icing for a children's party.

3 tbsp	cocoa powder, sifted	50 mL
2 tbsp	boiling water	25 mL
1¾ cups	all-purpose flour	425 mL
2 tsp	baking powder	10 mL
1 cup	soft margarine	250 mL
½ cup	sugar	125 mL
3	eggs, beaten	3
3 tbsp	skim milk	50 mL
1 tsp	vanilla extract	5 mL

Preheat oven to 350°F (180°C). Grease a 9 x 9 inch (23 x 23 cm) baking pan and line the bottom with waxed paper. Stir the cocoa powder and the boiling water together until smooth.

Sift the flour and baking powder together and beat in the cocoa mixture with the margarine, sugar, eggs, milk and vanilla. Beat until smooth. Spoon into prepared pan. Bake 25 to 30 minutes or until top springs back when pressed. Cool in the pan, before turning out on to a wire rack to cool completely. Makes 20 squares.

PER SERVING: ¹⁄₂₀ of recipe

1 ▢ + 2½ ▲ + 1 ++

Calories	194
g protein	3
g carbohydrate	18
g dietary fiber	1
g fat–total	13
g saturated fat	2
mg cholesterol	40
mg sodium	164

Cherry and Raisin Cake

A light fruit cake that is delicious as an afternoon snack—or serve with a cup of tea.

4 oz	glacé cherries, rinsed and dried	120 g
¾ cup	raisins	175 mL
¾ cup	soft margarine	175 mL
¼ cup	sugar	50 mL
1¼ cups	all-purpose flour	300 mL
¾ cup	whole-wheat flour	175 mL
1 tsp	baking powder	5 mL
3	eggs, beaten	3
	Grated peel and juice of 1 lemon	
3 tbsp	skim milk	50 mL

Preheat oven to 350°F (180°C). Grease an 8-inch (20-cm) cake pan and line bottom with waxed paper. Coarsely chop the cherries and mix together with the raisins and ⅓ of the flours.

Beat the margarine and sugar together until pale and creamy. Add the eggs and beat well. Beat in remaining flour and baking powder. Stir in the cherry mixture, lemon peel and juice, and milk. Spoon into a lightly greased and base-lined round 8-inch (20-cm) cake pan and level the top. Bake 50 to 60 minutes or until a skewer inserted into the center of the cake comes out clean. Allow to cool in the pan 10 minutes before turning out on to a wire rack to cool completely. Makes 12 to 16 servings.

PER SERVING: ½ of recipe

2 ▢ + ½ ✱ + 2½ ▲

Calories	271
g protein	5
g carbohydrate	36
g dietary fiber	2
g fat–total	13
g saturated fat	2
mg cholesterol	53
mg sodium	155

Spiced Apple and Almond Cake

This cake keeps for up to 3 days but it is suitable for freezing. For a more festive look, serve with a dollop of whipped cream or frozen whipped topping.

1 lb	Granny Smith apples (about 3), peeled, cored and coarsely chopped	500 g
1 tbsp	lemon juice	15 mL
3 tbsp	water	50 mL
1½ cups	all-purpose flour	375 mL
½ cup	whole-wheat flour	125 mL
2 tsp	baking powder	10 mL
1 tsp	baking soda	5 mL
½ cup	soft margarine	125 mL
½ cup	packed light brown sugar	125 mL
2	eggs, beaten	2
½ tsp	almond extract	2 mL
¼ cup	chopped almonds	60 mL
¼ tsp	ground cloves	1 mL
1 tsp	ground cinnamon	5 mL
½ tsp	ground nutmeg	2 mL
¼ cup	milk	60 mL

Preheat oven to 350°F (180°C). Grease an 8-inch (20-cm) round cake pan and line the bottom. Place all ingredients in a food processor or mixer bowl. Blend for a few seconds until thoroughly combined. Spoon the batter into prepared pan.

Bake 50 to 60 minutes or until a skewer inserted in the center comes out clean. Cool in the pan 10 minutes before turning out on to a wire rack to cool completely. Cut into slices. Makes 16 slices.

PER SERVING: ¹⁄₁₆ of recipe

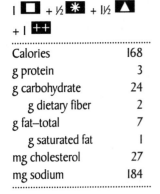

Calories	168
g protein	3
g carbohydrate	24
g dietary fiber	2
g fat–total	7
g saturated fat	1
mg cholesterol	27
mg sodium	184

German Plum Coffeecake

The plums' deep-red color is very attractive. You can also use apples,
peaches or apricots. Delicious served warm or cold.

⅓ cup	soft margarine	75 mL
1	egg	1
½ cup	milk	125 mL
1 tbsp	baking powder	15 mL
2 tbsp	sugar	25 mL
2 cups	all-purpose flour	500 mL
1 tsp	vanilla extract	5 mL
1 lb	fresh plums, cut in eighths	500 g
1 tbsp	sugar	15 mL
1 tsp	ground cinnamon	5 mL
¼ tsp	ground nutmeg	1 mL

Preheat oven to 400°F (200°C). Grease an 9-inch (23-cm) square
baking pan.

Beat together margarine, egg and milk. Stir in baking powder, 2
tbsp (25 mL) sugar , flour and vanilla.

Spoon mixture into prepared pan. Press plum pieces into dough,
making a pretty pattern. Combine 1 tbsp (15 mL) sugar, cinnamon
and nutmeg. Sprinkle over plums. Bake 30 to 35 minutes. Cool at
least 10 minutes before serving. Makes 16 servings.

PER SERVING: ⅟₁₆ of recipe

1 ☐ + ½ ◩ + 1 ▲

Calories	125
g protein	3
g carbohydrate	19
g dietary fiber	1
g fat–total	5
g saturated fat	1
mg cholesterol	14
mg sodium	111

Lemon Cake

A traditional cake enlivened with fresh lemon. For a little different flavor, substitute orange or grapefruit for the lemon peel.

❖ Best eaten within 1 to 2 days. Suitable for freezing. Store in an airtight container.

½ cup	soft margarine	125 mL
½ cup	sugar	125 mL
3	eggs	3
1½ cups	all-purpose flour	375 mL
1½ tsp	baking powder	7 mL
1 tbsp	finely grated lemon peel	15 mL
1 tsp	vanilla extract	5 mL

Preheat oven to 325°F (160°C). Grease a 9 x 5 inch (33 x 23 cm) loaf pan and line with waxed paper. Beat margarine and sugar until light and creamy. Beat in eggs, one at a time, beating well after each addition. Beat in flour, baking powder, lemon peel and vanilla. Spoon batter into prepared pan and level the top.

Bake about 1 hour or until a skewer inserted in center of cake comes out clean. Cool in the pan for a few minutes before turning out to cool on a wire rack. Makes 16 slices.

PER SERVING: ¹⁄₁₆ of recipe

1 ☐ + 1½ ▲

Calories	132
g protein	2
g carbohydrate	15
g dietary fiber	0
g fat–total	7
g saturated fat	1
mg cholesterol	40
mg sodium	99

Lemon and Almond Cake

The sliced lemons on top of the cake give an attractive finish. I found the combination of lemons and almonds very refreshing compared to traditional recipes of this type, which tend to be very sweet.

❖ Suitable for freezing.

1 cup	soft margarine	250 mL
½ cup	sugar	125 mL
3	eggs, beaten	3
1½ cups	all-purpose flour	375 mL
2 tsp	baking powder	10 mL
⅓ cup	ground almonds	75 mL
	Grated peel and juice of 1 large lemon	
½ tsp	almond extract	2 mL

To finish

2	lemons	2
1 tbsp	reduced-sugar marmalade	15 mL
1 tbsp	water	15 mL

Preheat oven to 325°F (160°C). Grease an 8-inch (20-cm) spring-form pan and line the bottom with waxed paper. Place all the cake ingredients in a large bowl. Beat with an electric mixer 2 to 3 minutes or until light and fluffy. Turn the mixture into prepared pan and smooth the top.

Pare entire peel and pith from lemons, then slice the flesh into thin rounds. Arrange on top of the cake.

Bake 50 to 60 minutes until golden and firm. Cool in the pan 5 minutes, then release the sides and cool on a wire rack. Warm marmalade and water together. Sieve and brush over the top of warm cake. Makes 14 to 16 slices.

PER SERVING: ¹⁄₁₄ of recipe

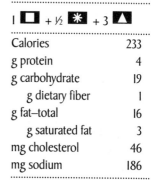

Calories	233
g protein	4
g carbohydrate	19
g dietary fiber	1
g fat–total	16
g saturated fat	3
mg cholesterol	46
mg sodium	186

Orange and Ginger Cookies

Sprinkle the cookies with a little granulated artificial sweetener when cooked if you prefer a sweeter taste.

❖ Best eaten within 1 to 2 days. Suitable for freezing.

½ cup	soft margarine	125 mL
¼ cup	sugar	60 mL
1	egg, beaten	1
1¼ cups	quick-cooking oats	300 mL
1 cup	all-purpose flour	250 mL
½ tsp	baking powder	2 mL
½ tsp	salt	2 mL
1 tbsp	ground ginger	15 mL
2 tsp	vanilla extract	10 mL
1 tbsp	orange extract	15 mL
2 tbsp	orange zest	25 mL
½ tbsp	milk (optional)	10 mL

Preheat oven to 375°F (190°C). Grease 2 baking sheets. Beat together margarine, sugar and egg. Add remaining ingredients and stir until combined, add milk if batter is too stiff. Drop mixture by heaping tablespoonfuls, about 2 inches (5 cm) apart on prepared baking sheets. Flatten slightly with a fork. Bake 12 to 15 minutes or until golden and just firm to the touch. Cool on a wire rack. Makes 24 cookies.

PER SERVING: ⅟₂₄ of recipe

½ ▢ + 1 ▲

Calories	67
g protein	1
g carbohydrate	7
g dietary fiber	0
g fat–total	4
g saturated fat	1
mg cholesterol	9
mg sodium	90

Date and Apricot Bars

These old-fashioned treats are a bit crumbly, and they're a hit with everyone in the family.

¾ cup	pitted dates, chopped	175 mL
⅔ cup	dried apricots, chopped	150 mL
½ cup	water	125 mL
1½ cups	all-purpose flour	375 mL
1⅓ cups	quick-cooking oats	325 mL
1 tsp	baking powder	5 mL
¼ cup	packed light brown sugar	60 mL
¾ cup	soft margarine	175 mL
1½ tsp	vanilla extract	7 mL

Place the dates and apricots in a saucepan with the water and simmer 10 minutes or until soft and the mixture forms a paste. Let cool.

Preheat oven to 375°F (190°C). Grease a 13 x 9 inch (33 x 23 cm) baking pan and line the bottom with waxed paper. Combine flour, oats, baking powder and sugar in a bowl. Cut in margarine and vanilla until mixture resembles coarse crumbs. Press half the mixture into the bottom of prepared pan. Spoon the date and apricot mixture over the top. Spoon the remaining oat mixture over to cover evenly and press down with your fingers. Bake 30 minutes or until lightly browned. Cool in the pan 10 minutes. Mark into 18 bars and cool completely on a wire rack. Makes 18 bars.

PER SERVING: ⅛ of recipe

½ ☐ + 1 ◪ + 1½ ▲

Calories	150
g protein	2
g carbohydrate	19
g dietary fiber	1
g fat–total	8
g saturated fat	1
mg cholesterol	0
mg sodium	92

Raisin Cookies

Younger children will enjoy making these cookies but may need some help from an adult to bake them, especially when they are handling hot equipment.

2 cups	all-purpose flour	500 mL
1 tsp	baking powder	5 mL
1 tsp	ground cinnamon	5 mL
1 tsp	allspice	5 mL
½ cup	soft margarine	125 mL
⅓ cup	sugar	75 mL
¾ cup	dried currants or raisins	175 mL
1	egg, beaten	1
1 tsp	vanilla extract	5 mL
5 tbsp	skim milk	75 mL

Preheat oven to 400°F (200°C). Grease a baking sheet. Place the flour, baking powder and cinnamon in a bowl. Cut in the margarine until the mixture looks like bread crumbs. Stir in the sugar and the currants or raisins. Combine the egg, vanilla and milk in a small bowl and beat together with a fork. Pour into the currant mixture in the bowl. Mix well. The mixture will be sticky.

Drop cookie dough in 14 spoonfuls 2 inches apart on the baking sheet. Bake 10 to 15 minutes or until golden brown. Cool on a wire rack. Makes 14 cookies.

RIGHT: *Red Pepper, Basil and Tuna Pasta Salad (page 28)*

PER SERVING: ¼ of recipe

1 ☐ + ½ ◪ + ½ ✳ + 1½ ▲

Calories	171
g protein	3
g carbohydrate	25
g dietary fiber	1
g fat–total	7
g saturated fat	1
mg cholesterol	15
mg sodium	94

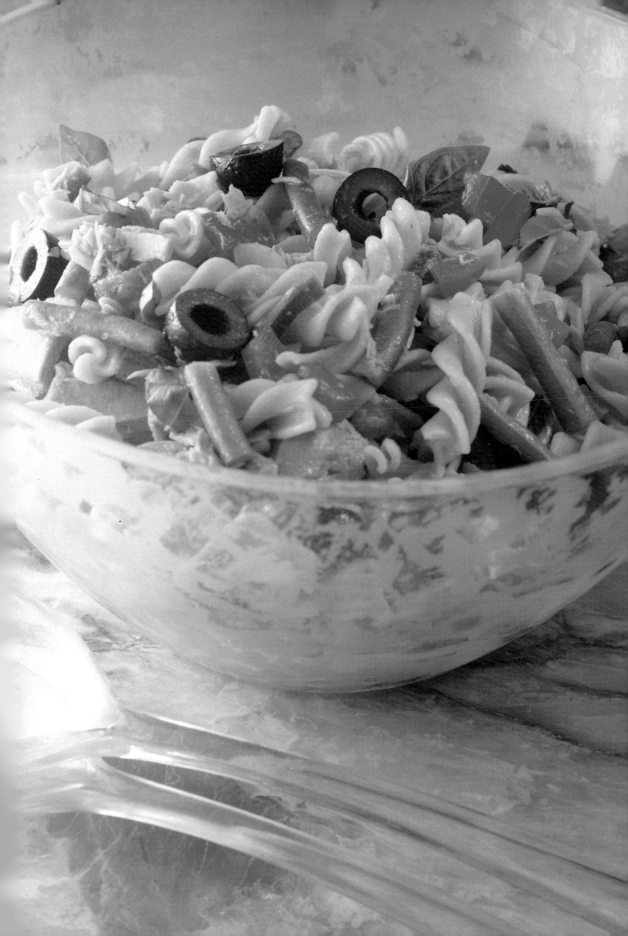

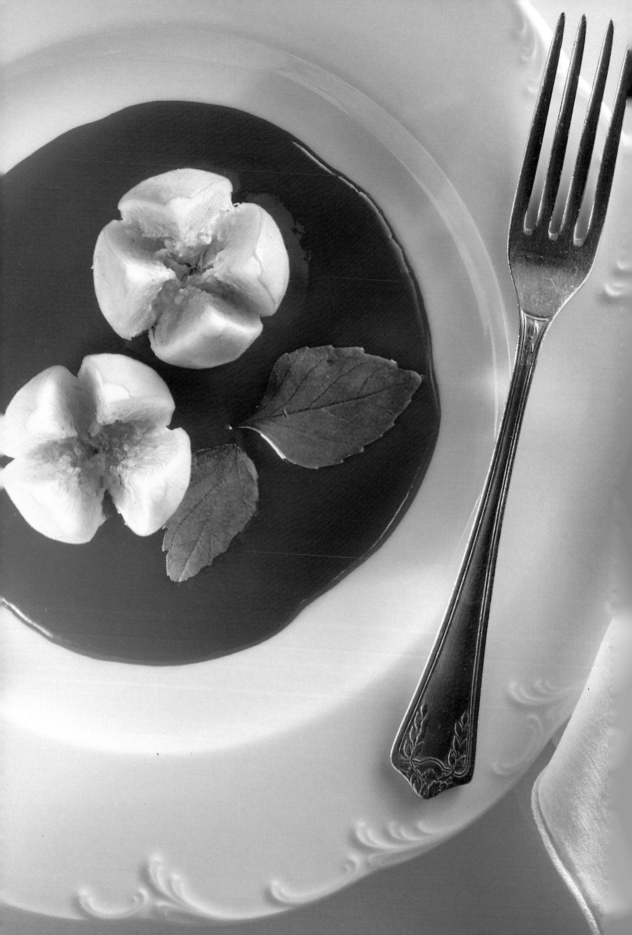

Tropical Island Cookies

If you prefer, substitute 4 tsp (20 mL) of orange or lemon peel for the extract.

2 cups	all-purpose flour	500 mL
2 tsp	baking powder	10 mL
½ cup	sugar	125 mL
1½ cups	shredded coconut	375 mL
1	whole egg, lightly beaten	1
1	egg white, lightly beaten	1
4 tsp	rum extract	20 mL
⅓ cup	soft margarine	75 mL

Preheat oven to 400°F (200°C). Grease a baking sheet. Combine the flour, baking powder, sugar and coconut in a bowl. Gradually add the egg, extract and margarine to the flour mixture and mix to a firm dough. (You may not need to add all of the margarine.)

Shape the cookie dough into 24 round balls and place 2 inches apart on the baking sheet. Bake 10 to 15 minutes or until golden brown. Cool on a wire rack. Makes 24 cookies.

LEFT: *Figs with Blackberry Sauce (page 146)*

PER SERVING: ¼ of recipe

❑ + ▲	
Calories	110
g protein	2
g carbohydrate	15
g dietary fiber	1
g fat–total	5
g saturated fat	2
mg cholesterol	9
mg sodium	74

Yellow Cake

This is a versatile cake that can be used as the basis for so many recipes, from elaborate birthday cakes to simple cupcakes. You can add many different flavors, such as cocoa powder, lemon or orange peel or coffee.

½ cup	soft margarine	125 mL
⅔ cup	sugar	150 mL
2	eggs, separated	2
1¾ cups	cake flour, sifted	425 mL
2 tsp	baking powder	10 mL
¼ tsp	salt	1 mL
½ tsp	vanilla extract	2 mL
½ cup	skim milk	125 mL

Preheat oven to 375°F (190°C). Grease two 9-inch (23-cm) cake pans and line bottoms with waxed paper. Beat margarine and sugar together until creamy. Beat in egg yolks, one at a time. Sift together flour, baking powder and salt. Beat into creamed mixture alternately with milk. Beat egg whites until stiff but not dry. Fold into cake batter. Divide batter between prepared pans.

Bake in the center of the oven about 25 minutes or until golden and firm to the touch. Turn out and cool on a wire rack. Makes 2 layers, 8 to 10 servings.

❖ Store in an airtight container. Best eaten within 2 to 3 days. Suitable for freezing.

TIP

❖ If using pure-fruit spread or reduced-sugar jam to fill the cake, remember to add the extra carbohydrate and calories.

❖ A pretty finishing touch is to sift a little granulated sweetener over a paper doily on top of the cake. When the doily is lifted, it leaves a lacy pattern.

PER SERVING: ⅛ of recipe

1½ ▢ + 1½ ✳ + 2½ ▲

Calories	273
g protein	4
g carbohydrate	37
g dietary fiber	0
g fat–total	12
g saturated fat	3
mg cholesterol	54
mg sodium	279

Desserts

I've tried to use artificial sweeteners wherever possible for these recipes to cut down on the sugar or carbohydrate content. Sweeteners are also useful to sweeten drinks and sweet sauces, such as custard.

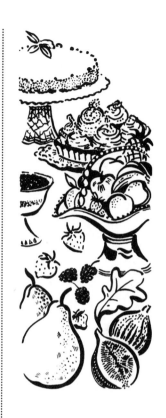

Old-Fashioned Baked Custard Tart

An old-fashioned dessert that is delicious served chilled.

½ cup	all-purpose flour	125 mL
½ cup	whole-wheat flour	125 mL
	Pinch of salt	
¼ cup	soft margarine	60 mL
1	egg yolk	1
2 tbsp	cold water	25 mL
3 tbsp	sugar	50 mL
4	eggs, lightly beaten	4
1½ cups	skim milk	375 mL
1 tsp	freshly grated nutmeg	5 mL

Sift the flours and salt into a bowl. Add any bran remaining in the sifter back into the bowl. Cut in the margarine until the mixture resembles fine bread crumbs. Add egg yolk and enough cold water to mix to a soft dough. Shape into a ball, cover and refrigerate 30 minutes.

Roll out pastry on a lightly floured surface and use to line an 8-inch (20-cm) flan or pie pan. Chill 15 to 20 minutes. Preheat oven to 425°F (220°C). Line pastry with foil and fill with dried beans and bake 5 minutes. Remove foil and beans and bake another 5 minutes.

Lightly whisk the sugar and eggs together. Heat the milk and half the nutmeg in a saucepan over low heat until warm. Add to the egg mixture. Strain the mixture and pour into the pastry shell. Sprinkle with the remaining nutmeg.

Bake 8 minutes. Reduce the temperature setting to 350°F (180°C) and bake another 15 to 20 minutes or until the pastry is golden and the custard is set. Cool on a wire rack. Serve cold. Makes 8 servings.

PER SERVING: ⅛ of recipe

1 ☐ + ½ ✳ + ½ ⊘ + 1½ ▲

Calories	181
g protein	7
g carbohydrate	19
g dietary fiber	1
g fat–total	9
g saturated fat	2
mg cholesterol	136
mg sodium	176

Apple Pie in Walnut Pastry

The pastry has a lovely nutty flavor, which complements the apples well. It is a fairly soft pastry and therefore needs to be chilled before rolling. Depending on your taste, you may prefer not to sweeten the apples with sweetener or you could sprinkle a little extra sweetener over the top of the pie after baking.

Pastry

½ cup	whole-wheat flour	125 mL
½ cup	all-purpose flour	125 mL
	Pinch of salt	
¼ cup	soft margarine	60 mL
½ cup	walnuts, very finely chopped	125 mL

Filling

2 lb	apples	1 kg
2 to 3 tbsp	granulated artificial sweetener	25 to 50 mL
½ tsp	ground cinnamon	2 mL
	Beaten egg to glaze	

Sift the flours and salt into a bowl. Add any bran remaining in the sifter back into the bowl. Cut in the margarine until the mixture resembles fine bread crumbs. Add the walnuts and enough cold water to mix to a soft dough. Shape into a ball, cover and refrigerate 30 minutes. Meanwhile, peel, core and slice the apples and layer with the sweetener to taste and spice in a deep 8-inch (20-cm) pie pan.

Preheat oven to 425°F (220°C). Roll out the pastry on a lightly floured board and cut a strip to cover the rim of the dish. Brush the rim with water and press the pastry down well. Dampen the pastry edge with water. Arrange remaining pastry over apples. Press down well and trim the edges. Reroll the trimmings and cut into leaves. Moisten with water and arrange on the pie. Glaze the pastry with a little beaten egg. Bake the pie 25 to 30 minutes or until the crust is golden and the apples are tender. Cover with foil if the crust browns too quickly. Serve hot or cold. Makes 8 servings.

PER SERVING: ⅛ of recipe

1 ▢ + 1 ◩ + 2½ ▲

Calories	229
g protein	4
g carbohydrate	30
g dietary fiber	4
g fat–total	12
g saturated fat	2
mg cholesterol	27
mg sodium	95

Lemon and Raisin Cheesecake

This baked cheesecake has a lovely lemon flavor which complements the raisins. I use an aspartame-based sweetener, which is not normally recommended for baking, but is very successful here and tastes sweet enough.

5 oz	golden raisins	150 g
	Finely grated peel and juice of 3 lemons	
¾ cup	all-purpose flour	175 mL
¾ cup	whole-wheat flour	175 mL
¼ cup	soft margarine	60 mL
2 to 3 tbsp	water	25 to 50 mL
1 tbsp	cornstarch	15 mL
2	8-oz (250 g) pkgs. fat free cream cheese, softened	2
2 to 3 tbsp	granulated artificial sweetener	25 to 50 mL
3	eggs, beaten	3
1 tsp	vanilla extract	5 mL

Place the raisins, lemon peel and juice in a bowl and let stand 30 minutes. Sift the flours into a bowl. Add any bran remaining in the sifter back into the bowl. Cut in the margarine until the mixture resembles fine bread crumbs. Add enough cold water to mix to a soft dough. Shape into a ball, cover and refrigerate 30 minutes.

Roll out pastry on a lightly floured surface to line the bottom and sides of a 9-inch (23-cm) round, tart pan with a removable bottom. Chill 15 minutes. Preheat oven to 400°F (200°C). Line pastry with foil and fill with dried beans and bake 5 minutes. Remove the foil and beans and bake another 5 minutes. Reduce the oven temperature to 325°F (160°C).

Beat the cornstarch, cream cheese, sweetener, eggs, vanilla, raisins and lemon juice together in a large bowl. Mix thoroughly. Pour the mixture into pastry shell and bake 45 minutes or until firm and golden. Allow to cool. Run a knife around the edge and remove . Chill before serving. Sprinkle with a little sweetener to serve, if desired. Makes 10 servings.

PER SERVING: ¹⁄₁₀ of recipe

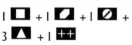

Calories	294
g protein	9
g carbohydrate	30
g dietary fiber	3
g fat–total	18
g saturated fat	7
mg cholesterol	96
mg sodium	407

Pineapple and Lemon Cheesecake

A light, refreshing cheesecake with a pleasing pineapple flavor.

¼ cup	soft margarine	60 mL
1 cup	finely crushed vanilla wafer crumbs	250 mL
1	8-oz (250 mL) can pineapple pieces in natural juice	1
1	envelope unflavored gelatin	1
1	8-oz (250 g) pkg. fat-free cream cheese, softened	1
⅔ cup	plain fat-free yogurt	150 mL
	Grated peel and juice of 1 small lemon	
3 tbsp	granulated artificial sweetener, or to taste	50 mL
2	egg whites	2

Melt the margarine in a small saucepan and stir in the crushed cookies until thoroughly mixed. Spread over the bottom of a 9-inch (23-cm) round pan with a removable bottom. Chill in the refrigerator until required. Drain the pineapple and reserve the juice and 4 pieces.

Pour the reserved juice into a small bowl. Sprinkle the gelatin over the juice and let stand 5 minutes to soften. Stand the bowl over a pan of hot water and stir until the gelatin has dissolved. Set aside to cool slightly. Place the soft cheese, yogurt, lemon rind and juice in a food processor or blender. Blend until smooth, then pour into a bowl. Add the pineapple to the processor and blend a few seconds until finely chopped, but not a purée. Stir into the cheese mixture with sweetener to taste. Whisk the egg whites until stiff peaks form. Lightly fold the gelatin into the pineapple mixture and lastly fold in the egg whites. Pour the mixture over the crumb base and refrigerate until set. Decorate with the reserved pineapple before serving. Makes 8 servings.

USING GELATIN

❖ Always add gelatin to liquid and not the other way round. When you are adding the dissolved gelatin to the mixture, there should not be a big temperature difference between the two. Never over-heat gelatin; if it gets too hot it will not set.

PER SERVING: ⅛ of recipe

½ ▢ + ½ ▱ + ½ ✳
+ 1 ⬛ + 2 ▲

Calories	212
g protein	6
g carbohydrate	17
g dietary fiber	1
g fat–total	14
g saturated fat	5
mg cholesterol	27
mg sodium	349

Strawberry Creams

I have made this recipe using a low-fat evaporated milk that I chilled overnight, and it gave a similar result with no difference in taste. If you can buy the low-fat evaporated milk, it will be about half the amount of fat per serving.

1	0.35-oz (10 g) pkg. sugar-free strawberry gelatin dessert	1
1 cup	boiling water	250 mL
1	12-oz (350 mL) can evaporated low-fat or whole milk, chilled overnight	1
	Sliced fresh strawberries and mint sprigs to decorate	

Dissolve the gelatin dessert in the boiling water in a medium bowl. Set aside until cooled. Meanwhile, using an electric mixer, beat the evaporated milk in a chilled bowl until thickened and doubled in volume. Fold the cooled gelatin mixture into the milk until thoroughly blended. Pour into 4 (1 cup/250 mL) dessert molds or individual dishes. It won't all fit at first but, as the mixture settles, top up with the remaining mixture. Chill about 3 hours or until set. Dip the molds in hot water 10 seconds and gently turn out on serving plates. Decorate with sliced fresh strawberries and mint sprigs. Makes 4 servings.

MANDARIN CREAMS

❖ When strawberries are not in season, substitute an orange gelatin dessert mix and decorate with a well-drained can of mandarin orange segments in natural juice.

PER SERVING: ¼ of recipe

½ ▰ + 1 ◆ 2% + ½ ▱

Calories	93
g protein	8
g carbohydrate	12
g dietary fiber	0
g fat–total	2
g saturated fat	1
mg cholesterol	7
mg sodium	150

Rhubarb and Ginger Fool

Ginger adds spicy flavor to this easy dessert. It is low in calories and fat.

1 lb	rhubarb, trimmed and cut into chunks	500 g
1 tbsp	finely grated fresh ginger	15 mL
3 tbsp	water	50 mL
3 to 4 tbsp	granulated artificial sweetener	50 to 60 mL
1 cup	skim milk	250 mL
2 tbsp	cornstarch	25 mL
1 tsp	vanilla extract	5 mL

Place the rhubarb, ginger and water into a saucepan over low heat. Cover and simmer 5 to 10 minutes or until soft. Cool. Reserve 4 pieces of rhubarb for decoration, and stir in 2 to 3 tbsp (25 to 50 mL) of the sweetener.

Combine a little of the milk with the cornstarch in a small saucepan; stir in remaining milk. Cook, stirring, over medium-low heat until very thick. Remove from the heat and stir in the vanilla and 1 tbsp (15 mL) of the sweetener. Fold the rhubarb into the custard and spoon into 4 individual glasses. Cover and refrigerate until chilled. Decorate with the reserved rhubarb before serving. Makes 4 servings.

PER SERVING: ¼ of recipe

½ ▱ + ½ ◆ Skim +
1 ++

Calories	63
g protein	3
g carbohydrate	12
g dietary fiber	2
g fat–total	0
g saturated fat	0
mg cholesterol	1
mg sodium	36

Tiramisu

This Italian delicious dessert is a favorite in Italian restaurants, but my recipe has fewer calories!

❖ Tirami Su, as the Italians would write it, literally means "pick me up." If you like the creamy dessert but don't like coffee, make a chocolate version instead. Use a chocolate liqueur and replace the strong coffee with a low-calorie chocolate drink.

1	egg, separated	1
2 tbsp	granulated artificial sweetener	25 mL
½ tsp	vanilla extract	2 mL
3	3-oz (75 g) pkgs. fat-free cream cheese, softened	3
½ cup	strong black coffee	125 mL
2 tbsp	coffee liqueur	25 mL
½	Yellow Cake layer (page 130)	½
½ tsp	cocoa powder	2 mL

Place the egg yolk, sweetener, vanilla extract and cream cheese in a bowl and beat to a smooth consistency. Whisk the egg white until stiff and gently fold into the cream cheese mixture with a spatula. Mix the coffee and liqueur together in a bowl. Cut the cake into 1-inch (2.5-cm) strips and dip into the coffee and liqueur until it absorbs the mixture, but not until it falls apart.

Layer half the cake in the bottom of 4 individual glass dishes or 1 medium serving dish, cutting into smaller pieces to fit. Cover with half the cheese mixture. Top with remaining cake and finish with a layer of cheese mixture. Dust with cocoa powder and refrigerate at least 1 hour before serving. Makes 4 servings.

PER SERVING: ¼ of recipe

1 ☐ + 2½ ✳ + 1 ⊘ + 3 ▲ + 1 ++

Calories	366
g protein	8
g carbohydrate	42
g dietary fiber	0
g fat–total	18
g saturated fat	5
mg cholesterol	120
mg sodium	428

Banana Cream Pie

It takes about 10 minutes to thicken the custard, so you'll need some patience. Because the meringue is made with less sugar, it will be slightly softer than a standard recipe, but it is still as nice.

❖ Best eaten the same day.

1	recipe Pastry for Normandy Apple Flan (page 161)	1
2	eggs, separated	2
2 tbsp	cornstarch	25 mL
1 tbsp	soft margarine	15 mL
1 cup	skim milk	250 mL
2 tbsp	granulated artificial sweetener or to taste	25 mL
1 tsp	vanilla extract	5 mL
2	medium bananas, sliced and tossed with lemon juice	2
3 tbsp	sugar	50 mL

Prepare pastry, chill and use to line an 8-inch (20-cm) tart pan. Chill 15 minutes in the refrigerator. Preheat oven to 425°F (220°C). Line pastry with foil and fill with dried beans and bake 5 minutes. Remove the foil and beans and bake another 10 minutes or until golden brown.

Beat the egg yolks, cornstarch and margarine in a heatproof bowl, until pale in color. Bring the milk almost to a boil in a saucepan, then gradually whisk into the egg mixture. Place the bowl over a pan of simmering water and cook, stirring constantly, until thick. Remove from the heat and allow to cool slightly. Stir in the sweetener and vanilla extract.

Arrange the banana slices in the bottom of the pastry shell, reserving a few for decoration. Pour the custard over the banana slices. Beat the egg whites until soft peaks form. Slowly beat in the sugar until stiff but not dry. Spoon the meringue over the custard, leaving the center uncovered. Bake at 300°F (180°C) 15 to 20 minutes or until the meringue is golden. Arrange the remaining banana slices in the center. Serve cold. Makes 8 servings.

PER SERVING: ⅛ of recipe

1½ ▢ + ½ ◢ + ½ ✳
+ ½ ⬗ + 2 ▲

Calories	244
g protein	6
g carbohydrate	32
g dietary fiber	2
g fat–total	11
g saturated fat	2
mg cholesterol	54
mg sodium	149

Apple and Blackberry Sponge Pudding

I don't add sugar or a sweetener to fresh fruit when making desserts, because I find that the fruit is sweet enough. However sweetener is given as an option in the recipe if you prefer to add it. Using raspberries in place of the blackberries makes a nice variation.

1 lb	apples, peeled, cored and sliced	500 g
8 oz	blackberries, rinsed	250 g
2 to 3 tbsp	granulated artificial sweetener or to taste	25 to 50 mL
5 tbsp	sugar	75 mL
¼ cup	soft margarine	60 mL
¼ cup	all-purpose flour	60 mL
½ tsp	baking powder	2 mL
	Grated peel and juice of 1 lemon	
1	egg, separated	1
½ cup	2 percent milk	125 mL
2 tbsp	sliced almonds	25 mL
	A little granulated artificial sweetener to serve (optional)	

Preheat oven to 350°F (180°C). Place the apples and blackberries in the bottom of a 1-quart (1-L) baking dish and sprinkle with the sweetener. Beat the sugar and margarine together in a medium bowl until creamy. Stir in the flour, baking powder, lemon peel and juice, egg yolk and milk and beat until smooth. (The mixture may look curdled.)

Whisk the egg white until stiff but not dry and fold into the mixture. Spoon over the apples and blackberries to cover. Sprinkle with the almonds. Place the dish in a roasting pan and add boiling water halfway up the side of the dish.

Bake 50 minutes or until the top is golden. Dust with a little granulated sweetener before serving if desired. Serve hot. Makes 6 servings.

PLUM SPONGE PUDDING

❖ Replace the apple and blackberries with 1½ lb (750 g) of ripe plums. Cut them in half and remove the pit before putting them in the dish. You probably will need very little, if any, sweetener.

PER SERVING: ⅙ of recipe

2 ▢ + 1 ✴ + 2 ◣

Calories	226
g protein	3
g carbohydrate	32
g dietary fiber	3
g fat–total	10
g saturated fat	2
mg cholesterol	37
mg sodium	121

Pears with Raspberry Sauce

This dessert is made even more attractive if you choose nicely shaped and evenly sized pears. Lay them sideways in the saucepan during cooking and turn occasionally so that they are evenly colored.

4	medium pears	4
1 cup	dry red wine	250 mL
1 or 2	cinnamon sticks	1 or 2
4	whole cloves	4
1 tbsp	lemon juice	15 mL
8 oz	raspberries, defrosted if frozen	250 g
2 tbsp	granulated artificial sweetener or to taste	25 mL

Peel the pears thinly, leaving the stems intact. Remove the core with a knife or apple corer and cut a small piece from the bottom of each pear so they can stand up.

Place the pears, wine, cinnamon, cloves and lemon juice in a medium saucepan over medium heat. Bring to a boil. Reduce heat, cover and simmer 15 minutes, basting and turning the pears so they are evenly colored. Remove from the heat and set aside.

To make the sauce, cook the raspberries about 5 minutes over low heat or until the raspberries are soft. Press the raspberries through a fine strainer to remove seeds. Stir the sweetener into the raspberries to taste. Drain the pears and mix 5 tbsp (75 mL) of the wine mixture with the raspberry mixture. Pour the sauce on to serving plates and add the pears. Decorate with fresh mint. Makes 4 servings.

PER SERVING: ¼ of recipe

2½ ◢ + 1 ▲ + 1 ++

Calories	168
g protein	1
g carbohydrate	33
g dietary fiber	6
g fat–total	1
g saturated fat	0
mg cholesterol	0
mg sodium	3

Summer Fruit Layers

This dessert takes time to prepare, but the result is impressive. Don't try to rush the gelatin layers. Make sure that each layer is chilled until completely set before adding another layer. Keep the remaining gelatin mixture at room temperature until required. The carbohydrate per serving is negligible. To frost glasses, rub the rim of the glasses with a lemon half and then dip in granulated artificial sweetener.

1	0.35-oz (10 g) pkg. sugar-free strawberry gelatin dessert	1
1 cup	boiling water	250 mL
1 cup	rosé wine	250 mL
4 oz	strawberries, hulled	120 g
4 oz	blueberries	120 g
4 oz	raspberries	120 g
1 cup	whipping cream	250 mL

Dissolve gelatin dessert in the boiling water in a medium bowl. Cool slightly, then stir in the wine. Cool to room temperature. Reserve 2 strawberries for decoration, slice remaining strawberries and arrange in the bottom of 8 small dessert glasses. Carefully pour a layer of the gelatin mixture over the strawberries. Chill in the refrigerator until set. Repeat with a layer of blueberries and gelatin mixture and chill until set. Finally, repeat with a layer of raspberries and gelatin mixture. Chill until firm.

Whip the cream until soft peaks form. Spoon a dollop of cream on each dessert. Top with a strawberry slice and serve. Serve with thin wafer cookies if desired. Makes 8 servings.

PER SERVING: ⅛ of recipe

½ ◪ + 3 ◮ + 1 ++

Calories	147
g protein	2
g carbohydrate	6
g dietary fiber	1
g fat–total	11
g saturated fat	7
mg cholesterol	41
mg sodium	41

Steamed Apple and Berry Pudding

Apples and blackberries are a classic combination, and now that frozen fruits are widely available, you can make this dessert any time.

1	medium apple, peeled, cored and sliced	1
2 tbsp	water	25 mL
8 oz	raspberries or blackberries, thawed if frozen	250 g
½ cup	soft margarine	125 mL
5 tbsp	sugar	75 mL
1 tsp	vanilla extract	5 mL
2	eggs, beaten	2
1⅓ cups	self-rising flour	325 mL
2 tbsp	hot water	25 mL

Lightly grease a 1-quart (1-L) nonmetal bowl. Simmer the apple with the water in a small saucepan until soft. Drain and arrange apples in the bottom of greased bowl with the raspberries or blackberries.

Beat the margarine and sugar together in a medium bowl until creamy. Add the vanilla extract and eggs, a little at a time, beating well after each addition. Stir in the flour and water to a stiff batter. Spoon over the fruit. Cover with greased waxed paper and foil and secure with string. Steam 1½ hours or until topping is cooked. Makes 8 to 10 servings.

PER SERVING: ⅛ of recipe

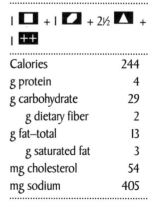

1 □ + 1 ◪ + 2½ ▲ + 1 ++

Calories	244
g protein	4
g carbohydrate	29
g dietary fiber	2
g fat–total	13
g saturated fat	3
mg cholesterol	54
mg sodium	405

RIGHT: *Chocolate Squares* (page 120)

PEACH AND RASPBERRY RICE

❖ Replace the apples and blackberries with fresh peaches and raspberries, or for a winter treat use canned peaches in natural juice and frozen raspberries and omit cooking the fruit.

PER SERVING: ¼ of recipe

1 ▢ + 1½ ◼ +
½ ◆ Skim

Calories	200
g protein	8
g carbohydrate	42
g dietary fiber	5
g fat–total	1
g saturated fat	0
mg cholesterol	3
mg sodium	89

Rice Pudding with Apple and Blackberry

Substitute fresh or frozen raspberries for the blackberries if they are not in season. If you use raspberries, you may not need as much sweetener, depending on your taste.

¼ cup	short-grain rice	60 mL
2 cups	skim milk	500 mL
	Finely grated peel and juice of 1 lemon	
1	vanilla bean, split open	1
3 tbsp	granulated artificial sweetener	50 mL
12 oz	apples, peeled, cored and sliced	350 g
8 oz	blackberries	250 g
⅔ cup	low-fat plain yogurt	150 mL

Place the rice, milk, lemon peel and vanilla bean in a medium saucepan over medium heat. Bring to a boil. Reduce heat and simmer, uncovered, stirring occasionally, until the rice is tender and most of the milk is absorbed, 30 to 40 minutes. Turn into a large bowl and stir in 1 tbsp (15 mL) of the sweetener. Let cool.

Meanwhile, place the apples and 2 tbsp (25 mL) of the lemon juice in a saucepan over low heat. Cover tightly and simmer until the apples are tender and still hold their shape. Add the blackberries and cook just a few seconds. Pour the fruit into a bowl. Stir in the remaining sweetener. Cool slightly, cover and refrigerate 1 hour. Fold the yogurt into the rice, cover and refrigerate 1 hour.

To serve, layer the apple and rice mixture in 4 individual glasses, discarding the vanilla bean. Top each with a blackberry and a slice of apple. Makes 4 servings.

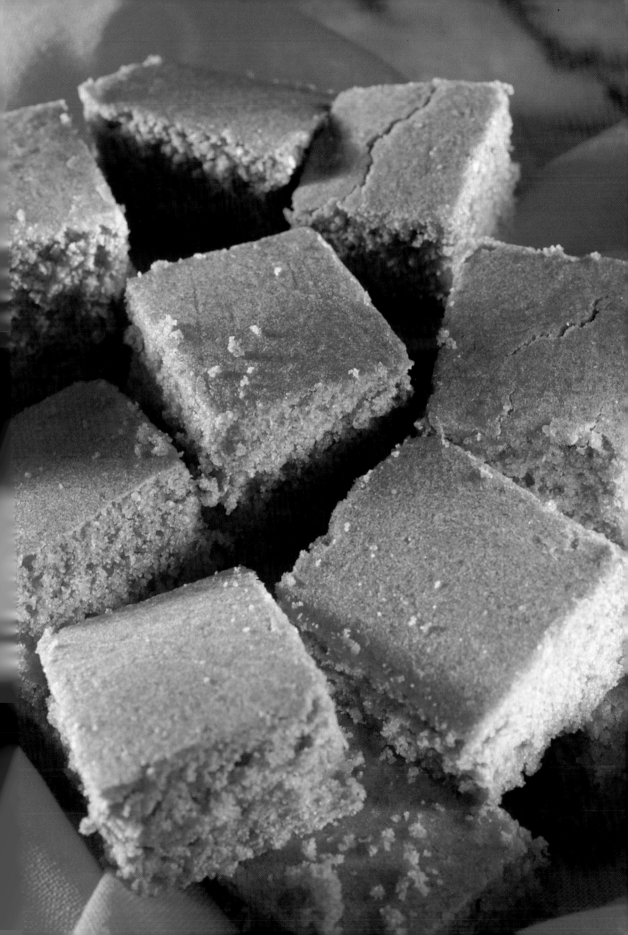

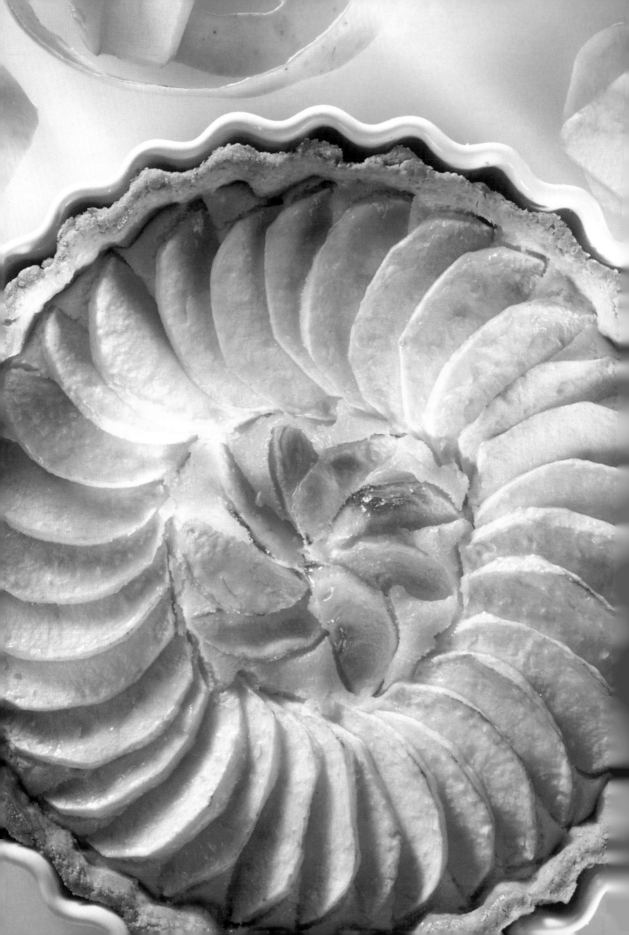

Spiced Apple Pie in Filo Pastry

Here is an apple pie that is low in fat and calories! Keep the fat content low by using only a small amount of melted soft margarine to brush the pastry before baking.

1 lb	apples, peeled, cored and sliced	500 g
¼ cup	water	60 mL
½ tsp	ground mixed spice	2 mL
½ tsp	ground cinnamon	2 mL
3 tbsp	golden raisins	50 mL
1 tbsp	granulated artificial sweetener	15 mL
1	sheet filo pastry	1
1 tbsp	soft margarine, melted	15 mL

Preheat oven to 425°F (220°C). Place the apples, water and spices in a small saucepan over low heat. Cook 5 minutes, stirring occasionally, or until soft. Stir in the raisins and sweetener and spoon into a small, shallow ovenproof dish.

Brush one side of the filo pastry with the melted margarine and then tear it into pieces. Arrange the filo pastry over the apple with the brushed side up. Bake 15 minutes or until the top is golden brown. Serve warm. Makes 4 servings.

LEFT: *Normandy Apple Flan (page 161)*

PER SERVING: ¼ of recipe

½ ☐ + 1½ ◰ + 1 ◢

Calories	130
g protein	1
g carbohydrate	26
g dietary fiber	3
g fat–total	4
g saturated fat	1
mg cholesterol	0
mg sodium	50

Figs with Blackberry Sauce

Depending on the sweetness of the blackberries, you may not need to add any sweetener. When figs are not available, serve this sauce on sliced peaches or melon.

❖ A perfect fig will be unblemished and will just yield when you hold it without pressing on it. It can be any color from pale green to purple.

8 oz	blackberries	250 g
2 tbsp	water	25 mL
1 tsp	arrowroot or cornstarch	5 mL
2 tsp	water	10 mL
1 to 2 tsp	granulated artificial sweetener (or to taste)	5 to 10 mL
8	ripe fresh figs	8

Place the blackberries and water in a small saucepan over low heat. Cook 2 to 3 minutes or until soft. Combine arrowroot or cornstarch and water. Stir mixture into the blackberries and boil, stirring, 1 minute to thicken.

Press the blackberries through a fine strainer to remove seeds. Stir in the sweetener to taste.

Cut off the fig stems. From the stem end, make 2 right-angle cuts in each fig, three-quarters of the way through. Open up to resemble flowers. Place 2 figs on each of 4 serving plates. Pour a little blackberry sauce over each fig. Serve the remaining sauce separately. Makes 4 servings.

PER SERVING: ¼ of recipe

2 ◼

Calories	106
g protein	1
g carbohydrate	27
g dietary fiber	6
g fat–total	1
g saturated fat	0
mg cholesterol	0
mg sodium	1

Chilled Lemon Soufflé

*I remember making my first lemon soufflé during my home economics
class. This recipe uses a granulated sweetener to reduce the sugar
content and also the calories.*

	Grated peel and juice of 3 lemons	
6	eggs, separated	6
5 tbsp	granulated artificial sweetener	75 mL
2 tbsp	unflavored gelatin powder	25 mL
1½ cups	whipping cream	375 mL
¼ cup	chopped mixed nuts, toasted	60 mL
	Shreds of lemon peel to decorate	

Tie a double strip of waxed paper around a 1-quart (1-L) soufflé
dish to make a 3-inch (7.5-cm) collar. Lightly brush the inside of
the paper with a little oil. Set aside.

With an electric mixer, beat the lemon peel, egg yolks and sweetener together in a bowl until pale. Pour 7 tbsp (115 mL) of the
lemon juice into a small saucepan, sprinkle in the gelatin and let
soak 5 minutes to soften. Place over low heat and stir until the
gelatin dissolves. Cool slightly, then stir into the egg yolk mixture.

Whip the cream in a medium bowl until it forms soft peaks.
Reserving a little for piping, fold the remaining cream into the egg
yolk mixture.

Beat the egg whites in a large bowl until stiff but not dry. With a
large spatula, carefully fold egg whites into the egg yolk mixture.
Gently pour the mixture into the prepared soufflé dish. Refrigerate
at least 4 hours or until set.

Carefully ease the paper collar away from the soufflé with a
knife dipped in hot water. Press the toasted nuts around the
edge of the soufflé with a small metal spatula. Decorate the top
with cream whirls and the lemon peel. Serve as soon as possible.
Makes 6 to 8 servings.

NOTE

❖ Raw eggs, and dishes
containing them, are unsuit-
able for older adults, young
children or pregnant women.

PER SERVING: ⅙ of recipe

½ ❋ + 1½ ⊘ + 5 ▲

Calories	321
g protein	10
g carbohydrate	4
g dietary fiber	1
g fat–total	30
g saturated fat	16
mg cholesterol	294
mg sodium	91

No-Sugar Custard Sauce

Sweeteners should generally be added after the custard is boiled because some types lose their sweetness at high temperatures.

1 cup	skim milk	250 mL
1 tbsp	cornstarch	15 mL
1 tsp	vanilla extract	5 mL
	Artificial sweetener to taste	

Combine a little of the milk with the cornstarch in a small saucepan; stir in remaining milk. Cook, stirring, over medium-low heat until thickened. Remove from the heat and stir in the vanilla and sweetener. Serve warm or chilled. Makes 1 cup (250 mL).

PER SERVING: ¼ cup (50 mL)

½ ◆ Skim

Calories	31
g protein	2
g carbohydrate	5
g dietary fiber	0
g fat–total	0
g saturated fat	0
mg cholesterol	1
mg sodium	32

Lemon and Lime Meringue Pie

A variation of a family favorite. Use an artificial sweetener instead of sugar in desserts such as this.

1	recipe Pastry for Normandy Apple Flan (page 161)	1
	Finely grated peel and juice of 1 small lemon	
	Finely grated peel and juice of 1 small lime	
1 tbsp	soft margarine	15 mL
3 tbsp	cornstarch	50 mL
2	eggs, separated	2
1 tbsp	granulated artificial sweetener or to taste	15 mL
2 tbsp	sugar	25 mL

Prepare pastry, chill and use to line an 8-inch (20-cm) tart pan. Chill 15 minutes in the refrigerator. Preheat oven to 425°F (220°C). Line pastry with foil and fill with dried beans and bake 5 minutes. Remove the foil and beans and bake another 10 minutes or until golden brown. Remove the paper and baking beans and bake another 10 minutes or until golden. Reduce the oven temperature to 300°F (150°C).

Meanwhile, prepare the filling. Pour the lemon and lime juices into a 1 cup (250 mL) measure. Add enough cold water to make 1 cup (250 mL). Combine a little of the juice mixture with the cornstarch in a small saucepan; stir in remaining juice mixture and margarine. Bring to a boil. Reduce heat and cook, stirring, over medium-low heat until thickened. Beat a little of lemon mixture into the egg yolks. Return to saucepan and cook, stirring, 1 minute. Cool slightly and add the sweetener to taste. Pour into the pastry shell.

Beat the egg whites until soft peaks form. Gradually beat in the sugar until stiff but not dry. Spoon the meringue over the filling. Bake 20 to 25 minutes or until golden brown. Serve warm or cold. Makes 8 servings.

NOTE

❖ Due to the reduced sugar content, the meringue topping will have a slightly softer texture.

PER SERVING: ⅛ of recipe

1½ ▮ + 2 ▲

Calories	203
g protein	4
g carbohydrate	23
g dietary fiber	2
g fat–total	11
g saturated fat	2
mg cholesterol	53
mg sodium	133

Nectarine and Raspberry Dessert

A low-fat dessert using fresh summer fruits. For a special finish, rub the rim of the sundae glasses with a lemon half and then coat with a granulated artificial sweetener before filling.

2	ripe nectarines	2
5 oz	raspberries, fresh or frozen	150 g
1	8-oz (250 g) pkg. light cream cheese, softened	1
¾ cup	fat free sugar-free raspberry yogurt	175 mL
3 tbsp	granulated artificial sweetener or to taste	50 mL
	Mint leaves to decorate	

Halve and remove seeds from the nectarines. Place in a blender or food processor and purée until smooth. Add a little sweetener to taste and set side. Reserving 4 raspberries for decoration, purée the remaining raspberries until smooth and strain through to remove the seeds, if desired. Pour into the bottom of four sundae dishes. Lightly fold the cheese and yogurt together, and add a little sweetener to taste.

Layer the yogurt mixture and nectarine purée in the sundae dishes, finishing with a layer of yogurt mixture. Chill before serving, decorated with the reserved raspberries and mint leaves. Makes 4 servings.

PER SERVING: ¼ of recipe

2½ ▱ + ½ ◆ Skim +
1 ▱ + 1½ ▲

Calories	262
g protein	11
g carbohydrate	32
g dietary fiber	2
g fat–total	10
g saturated fat	6
mg cholesterol	34
mg sodium	220

Frozen Orange Cups

I find it easier to scoop out the pulp using a sharp knife to score around the outside and a spoon to scoop it out. This very refreshing dessert and is particularly suitable for serving in the summer months.

4	large oranges	4
1¼ cups	low-fat plain yogurt	300 mL
1	8-oz (250 g) carton light cream cheese, softened	1
¼ cup	granulated artificial sweetener	60 mL
	Sprigs of fresh mint to decorate	

Trim a small amount from the bottom of each orange so that they stand upright. Cut away the stem ends and set aside. Scoop out the pulp and place in a food processor or blender with the yogurt and cream cheese. Add the sweetener and process 10 to 20 seconds or until smooth. Pass through a sieve if desired. Pour into a freezer-proof container. Freeze the orange cups and the orange mixture 4 hours, mashing the frozen mixture with a fork after 2 hours to remove ice crystals. (Or, you can process the mixture in the food processor or blender.) Remove the ice cream from the freezer 10 minutes before serving. Serve in scoops in the orange cups. Decorate with mint. Makes 4 servings.

PER SERVING: ¼ of recipe

2 ▱ + ½ ◆ Skim +
1½ ◿

Calories	156
g protein	14
g carbohydrate	25
g dietary fiber	2
g fat–total	0
g saturated fat	0
mg cholesterol	6
mg sodium	333

Lime Torte

I have to thank our friends Jo and Howard for this recipe. Jo made a dessert that used mascarpone cheese and I thought it must be possible to use a lower-fat cheese and to reduce the sugar content. It is still, however, quite high in calories and would be suitable for entertaining rather than as an everyday dessert.

1¼ cups	graham-cracker crumbs	300 mL
¼ cup	soft margarine, melted	60 mL
2	8-oz (250 g) pkgs. light cream cheese, softened	2
3 tbsp	granulated artificial sweetener Finely grated peel and juice of 2 limes Shredded peel of 1 lime to decorate	50 mL

Mix together the crumbs and margarine in a small bowl and press into the bottom of an 8-inch (20-cm) springform pan. Refrigerate 15 minutes.

Beat together the cream cheese, sweetener, grated lime peel and juice in a medium bowl until blended. Spread over the crumb crust. Cover and refrigerate at least 2 hours. Decorate with shredded lime peel before serving. Makes 6 to 8 servings.

PER SERVING: ⅙ of recipe

1½ ☐ + 1 ⊘ + 4 ▲

Calories	348
g protein	10
g carbohydrate	25
g dietary fiber	1
g fat–total	23
g saturated fat	10
mg cholesterol	42
mg sodium	445

Clafouti

Clafouti is a French dessert that I've adapted. I make this recipe when cherries are in season; otherwise, the dish can be rather expensive.

3 tbsp	all-purpose flour	50 mL
	A pinch of salt	
3	eggs, beaten	3
2 tbsp	sugar	25 mL
1½ cups	milk	375 mL
12 oz	fresh red cherries, pitted	350 g
2 tbsp	soft margarine	25 mL
2 tbsp	granulated artificial sweetener	25 mL

Preheat oven to 425°F (220°C). Sift together the flour and salt into a bowl, then beat in the eggs and sugar. Heat the milk until almost boiling and beat into the egg mixture.

Lightly grease a large, shallow ovenproof dish and arrange the cherries over the bottom. Pour the batter over the top and dot with the margarine.

Bake 20 to 25 minutes until the custard is set and golden brown. Sprinkle with the sweetener to taste and serve warm. Makes 8 servings.

❖ This dish is super made with pitted plums or prunes in place of the cherries.

PER SERVING: ⅛ of recipe

1 ◪ + ½ ✳ + ½ ◲ + 1 ◪

Calories	129
g protein	5
g carbohydrate	15
g dietary fiber	1
g fat–total	6
g saturated fat	2
mg cholesterol	83
mg sodium	106

Peach Yogurt Crunch

A simple dessert that children can easily make themselves, with the help of an adult to purée the peaches. Substitute other canned fruit, such as apricots, or pears, for a variation.

1	14-oz (398 mL) can peach slices in natural juice	1
3 tbsp	granulated artificial sweetener or to taste	50 mL
1 pint	fat-free frozen vanilla yogurt	500 mL
4	graham crackers	4

Drain the peaches, reserving the juice. Place the peaches and 2 tbsp (25 mL) of the juice in a blender or food processor and blend to a smooth purée. Stir in 2 tbsp (25 mL) of sweetener or to taste.

Layer the peach purée and yogurt in 4 or 5 glasses. Crumble the crackers over the top and serve. Make 4 or 5 servings.

PER SERVING: ¼ of recipe

1 ▰ + ½ ◆ Skim + 2½ ✳ + ½ ⬭

Calories	169
g protein	6
g carbohydrate	36
g dietary fiber	2
g fat–total	1
g saturated fat	0
mg cholesterol	2
mg sodium	111

Strawberry Milkshake

Make sure that the milk is ice-cold before you make the milkshake so that it can be served while it is frothy. Add a little artificial sweetener if you like to give a sweeter taste.

6 oz	fresh strawberries, hulled	175 g
1	6-oz (175 g) carton light strawberry yogurt	1
2 cups	skim milk	500 mL

Place all the ingredients in a blender and process for a few seconds until smooth and frothy. Pour into tall glasses and serve. Makes 4 servings.

PEACH MELBA SHAKE

❖ Use a large ripe peach and a carton of raspberry yogurt.

PER SERVING: ¼ of recipe

½ ◆ + 2 ◆ Skim

Calories	102
g protein	6
g carbohydrate	18
g dietary fiber	1
g fat–total	1
g saturated fat	0
mg cholesterol	5
mg sodium	84

Holiday Cooking

Holidays are meant to be enjoyed, so try to make everything as normal as possible for you and your family. With a little care and advance planning, you can enjoy holidays and stay in control of your diabetes. This chapter includes recipes for many traditional holiday foods. The whole family will like these dishes.

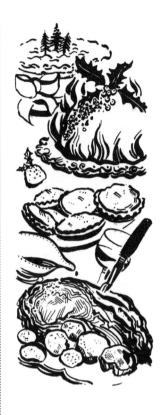

Cranberry Sauce

Fresh cranberries are usually available in supermarkets just before Christmas. Keep the sugar content low by using an artificial sweetener to sweeten the sauce.

❖ This sauce will not keep in a jar the way a high-sugar version will, but it will freeze successfully. Thaw thoroughly before serving.

1	12-oz (350 g) package fresh cranberries, picked over and rinsed	1
	Grated peel and juice of 1 orange	
5 tbsp	water	75 mL
2 to 3 tbsp	granulated artificial sweetener or to taste	25 to 50 mL

Place the cranberries, orange peel, orange juice and water in a saucepan over low heat. Simmer 15 minutes or until the berries are tender. Remove from the heat and add the sweetener to taste. Makes 6 to 8 servings.

PER SERVING: ⅙ of recipe

½ ◨

Calories	28
g protein	0
g carbohydrate	7
g dietary fiber	2
g fat–total	0
g saturated fat	0
mg cholesterol	0
mg sodium	1

Roast Rock Cornish Hens

Many people like to serve individual Rock Cornish hens at Christmas instead of turkey, particularly if the number of guests is small.

2 tbsp	olive oil	25 mL
4	Rock Cornish hens, thawed and rinsed	4
1	lemon sliced	1
	Sprigs of thyme	
	Bay leaves	
1 tbsp	all-purpose flour	15 mL
1 cup	chicken broth	250 mL
	Salt and freshly ground black pepper	

Preheat oven to 325°F (160°C). Heat the oil in a large Dutch oven over medium heat. Add the hens and cook, turning often, until browned. Place lemon slices, thyme and bay leaves in the cavity of each hen.

Cover and bake 1½ hours or until the hens are tender. Place the hens on a heated serving dish and keep hot. Meanwhile, skim the fat from the cooking juices. Stir in the flour and gradually add the stock. Boil, stirring constantly, 2 to 3 minutes and season with salt. Remove lemon slices and herbs before serving. Serve the gravy with the hens. Serve with wild rice and green vegetables. Makes 4 servings.

PER SERVING: ¼ of recipe

12 ⬛ + 2½ ◮ + 1 ➕➕

Calories	804
g protein	84
g carbohydrate	2
g dietary fiber	0
g fat–total	48
g saturated fat	13
mg cholesterol	268
mg sodium	1284

Peppered Roast Beef

Roast beef is ideal to serve on Christmas day instead of turkey. The spicy coating gives the beef a rich flavor.

TRADITIONAL SUNDAY
DINNER

❖ Fresh Leek Soup with Blue
Cheese (page 11)

❖ Peppered Roast Beef
served with Mini Yorkshire
Puddings (opposite)

❖ Dry-Roasted Potatoes
(page 168), carrots and a
green vegetable

❖ Apple Pie in Walnut
Pastry (page 133)

3½-lb	lean beef roast, such as eye of round	1.75 kg
3 tbsp	crushed mixed peppercorns	50 mL
6 tbsp	prepared horseradish sauce	100 mL
2 tbsp	all-purpose flour	25 mL
2 tbsp	cold water	25 mL
2 cups	beef stock	500 mL
	Salt and freshly ground black pepper	

Preheat oven to 425°F (220°C). Trim the beef of any excess fat and pat dry with paper towels. Mix the peppercorns and horseradish sauce together to form a paste. Spread the paste over the meat and place on a rack set in a roasting pan. Cover and cook 15 minutes per 1 lb (500 g), plus 15 minutes, for rare, 20 minutes per 1 lb (500 g), plus 20 minutes for medium, and 25 minutes per 1 lb (500 g), plus 25 minutes for well done.

Remove the roast from the oven and let stand, covered, on a warmed platter about 10 minutes before carving.

Drain the excess fat from the roasting pan. Mix the flour with the cold water to form a smooth paste. Stir the paste into the pan juices with the stock. Bring to a boil. Reduce heat and simmer, stirring constantly until the gravy is thickened. Season with salt and pepper.

Serve the roast beef with potatoes and green vegetables. Makes 8 servings.

PER SERVING: ⅛ of recipe

8½ 🚫 + 1 ➕➕

Calories	386
g protein	59
g carbohydrate	2
g dietary fiber	0
g fat–total	14
g saturated fat	6
mg cholesterol	141
mg sodium	238

Normandy Apple Flan

Even though I have adapted this dessert from the original, reducing the fat and calories, it is still rather high for an everyday meal. However, it does make a nice dessert when entertaining, or as an occasional treat. It is best served warm.

Pastry

¾ cup	all-purpose flour	175 mL
¾ cup	whole-wheat flour	175 mL
	A pinch of salt	
⅓ cup	soft margarine	75 mL
2 to 3 tbsp	cold water	25 to 50 mL

Filling

¼ cup	soft margarine	60 mL
2 tbsp	granulated artificial sweetener	25 mL
2	eggs	2
2 tbsp	cornstarch	25 mL
4 oz	ground almonds	120 g
¼ tsp	almond extract	1 mL
1¼ lb	apples	625 g
2 tbsp	reduced-sugar apricot jam	25 mL
2 tbsp	water	25 mL

Prepare the pastry: Sift the flours and salt into a bowl. Add any bran remaining in the sifter back into the bowl. Cut in the margarine until the mixture resembles fine bread crumbs. Add enough cold water to mix to a soft dough. Shape into a ball, cover and refrigerate 30 minutes.

Preheat oven to 400°F (200°C). Roll out dough on a lightly floured board to an 11-inch (28-cm) circle. Use to line a 9-inch (23-cm) tart pan. Line pastry with foil and add about 1½ cups (375 mL) dried beans. Bake 10 minutes. Remove the beans and foil and bake 5 minutes. Remove from oven.

PER SERVING: ⅛ of recipe

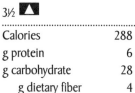

Calories	288
g protein	6
g carbohydrate	28
g dietary fiber	4
g fat–total	18
g saturated fat	3
mg cholesterol	43
mg sodium	140

Prepare the filling: Beat the margarine with the sweetener. Beat in the eggs, cornstarch, ground almonds and almond extract. Spread the almond mixture over the cooled pastry shell. Peel, core and thinly slice the apples. Arrange over the almond mixture. Bake 8 minutes. Reduce the heat to 350°F (180°C) and cook another 15 to 20 minutes or until golden.

Melt the apricot jam and water together in a small saucepan. Remove the tart from the pan and brush with the apricot glaze. Serve warm. Makes 8 servings.

Tropical Paradise Fruit Salad

Exotic fruits such as mango and lychee are now readily available from supermarkets or ethnic markets. This is a refreshing dessert that has no fat and is low in calories.

2	small oranges, peeled and segmented	2
2	kiwifruit, peeled and sliced	2
1	small pineapple, skin removed and diced	1
1	small mango, peeled, seed removed and diced	1
1	Galia melon, peeled and diced	1
4	lychees, skin and seeds removed, halved	4
½ cup	unsweetened orange juice	125 mL
½ cup	diet lemonade	125 mL
2 tbsp	rum (optional)	25 mL

Place all the fruit in a large bowl and toss lightly to mix. Add the orange juice, lemonade and rum, if using. Cover and chill 1 to 2 hours. Serve chilled. Makes 6 servings.

PINEAPPLE

❖ Some varieties of pineapple have a green skin when they are ripe. A pineapple is ripe when it has a rich pineapple fragrance.

PER SERVING: ⅙ of recipe

3 ◪

Calories	136
g protein	2
g carbohydrate	32
g dietary fiber	4
g fat–total	1
g saturated fat	0
mg cholesterol	0
mg sodium	8

Raspberry Trifle

A mixture of summer fruits may be used in place of the raspberries. For a burst of summer in the middle of winter, I use a package of frozen mixed berries.

½	1-lb (500 g) package frozen raspberries without sugar, thawed and drained	½
1	0.35-oz (10 g) package sugar-free raspberry gelatin dessert	1
2 tbsp	all-purpose flour	25 mL
1 cup	skim milk	250 mL
1 tsp	vanilla extract	5 mL
2 tbsp	granulated artificial sweetener or to taste	25 mL
½ cup	whipping cream, whipped, or a reduced-fat whipped topping	125 mL

Place the fruit in the bottom of a glass serving bowl. Prepare the gelatin dessert mix according to the directions on the package. Pour the mixture over the raspberries and place in the refrigerator to set.

Combine flour and 2 tbsp (25 mL) milk to a paste in a saucepan. Whisk in remaining milk. Cook, stirring constantly, over medium heat until thickened. Remove from the heat and add vanilla and artificial sweetener to taste. Allow to cool before pouring over the gelatin. Spread the whipped cream over the custard, cover and refrigerate until chilled. Makes 6 to 8 servings.

PER SERVING: ⅙ of recipe

1 �◻ + ½ ◢ + ½ ▲

Calories	105
g protein	4
g carbohydrate	15
g dietary fiber	4
g fat–total	4
g saturated fat	2
mg cholesterol	12
mg sodium	24

No-Added-Sugar Steamed Pudding

A moist pudding with no added sugar that still tastes rich and delicious.

1 cup	whole-wheat flour	250 mL
¼ tsp	salt	1 mL
½ tsp	ground nutmeg	2 mL
½ tsp	ground mixed spice	2 mL
½ cup	soft margarine	125 mL
2	eggs, beaten	2
	Grated peel and juice of 1 lemon	
2 tbsp	brandy	25 mL
1	small apple, cored and finely grated	1
2	large carrots, finely grated	2
2½ cups	soft whole-wheat bread crumbs	625 mL
2 oz	chopped mixed nuts	60 g
6 oz	dried currants	175 g
6 oz	dark raisins	175 g
8 oz	golden raisins	250 g

In a large bowl, sift together the flour, salt and spices, adding back any bran remaining in the sifter back into the bowl. Stir in all the remaining ingredients and mix well until thoroughly combined. Spoon into two 3-cup (750-mL) lightly greased pudding molds. Cover with a double thickness of buttered, pleated waxed paper, then with a layer of pleated foil. Secure with string.

Steam the puddings in a large steamer over a pan of gently simmering water 4½ hours. Let cool, then cover with fresh waxed paper and foil. Store in a cool, dry place for up to 2 weeks. To serve, steam 1½ to 2 hours or until heated through. Makes two 3-cup (750-mL) puddings or 20 servings.

❖ Serve with No-Sugar Custard Sauce (page 148) or Low-Sugar Rum or Brandy Sauce: Make as for Reduced-Sugar Custard and stir in 1 tbsp (15 mL) of brandy or rum and 1 tbsp (15 mL) soft margarine.

PER SERVING: ¹⁄₂₀ of recipe

1 ☐ + 1½ ◪ + 1½ ▲

Calories	213
g protein	5
g carbohydrate	34
g dietary fiber	3
g fat–total	7
g saturated fat	1
mg cholesterol	22
mg sodium	184

Creamy Fruit Dessert

This is an easy dessert to make yet looks impressive if set in a decorative jelly mold and decorated with fresh summer fruits. I like to serve this with strawberries, raspberries, red currants and black currants, grown in my mother's garden and full of flavor.

1 cup	boiling water	250 mL
1	0.35-oz (10 g) package sugar-free raspberry gelatin dessert	1
1	8-oz (250 g) package frozen mixed fruits or raspberries	1
1	1.3-oz (35 g) package whipped topping	1
½ cup	skim milk	125 mL
⅔ cup	raspberry-flavored nonfat yogurt	150 mL

Pour the boiling water into a medium bowl, add the gelatin dessert mix and stir to dissolve. Stir the frozen fruit into the gelatin mixture.

Prepare whipped topping with the milk according to the package instructions. Fold in the yogurt. Fold the yogurt mixture into the gelatin mixture. Cover and refrigerate 2 or 3 hours or until set. Makes 6 servings.

PER SERVING: ⅙ of recipe

1½ ▱ + ½ ◆ Skim
+ ½ ▲

Calories	110
g protein	4
g carbohydrate	19
g dietary fiber	1
g fat–total	3
g saturated fat	2
mg cholesterol	1
mg sodium	70

Mini Yorkshire Puddings

The perfect accompaniment to roast beef, Yorkshire pudding can count as a bread serving.

1 cup	all-purpose flour, sifted	250 mL
1	egg, beaten	1
1 cup	skim milk	250 mL
¼ cup	olive or sunflower oil	60 mL
	Salt and freshly ground black pepper	

Preheat oven to 425°F (220°C). Sift the flour into a bowl. Beat the egg and milk together. Make a well in the center of the flour and beat in the egg mixture until smooth. Allow the mixture to stand 15 minutes.

Divide the oil among cups in a 12-cup muffin pan in the oven a few minutes. Quickly pour the batter evenly into the muffin cups. Bake 20 to 25 minutes or until puffed and golden brown. Makes 12 servings.

Variation
Herbed Yorkshire Pudding
Add ½ tsp (2 mL) dried mixed herbs to the batter.

PER SERVING: ½ of recipe

½ ☐ + 1 ▲

Calories	91
g protein	2
g carbohydrate	9
g dietary fiber	0
g fat–total	5
g saturated fat	1
mg cholesterol	18
mg sodium	60

Dry-Roasted Potatoes

Roast potatoes without the fat! These potatoes are a mini-version of baked potatoes with a crunchy outside and soft potato in the center. They are best served with a roast dinner with gravy, otherwise they may seem rather dry.

2½ lb	Russet potatoes, peeled and halved	1.25 kg
	Salt	
2 tsp	ground paprika	10 mL

Preheat oven to 425°F (220°C). Cook the potatoes in lightly salted boiling water 10 minutes. Drain well and turn into a roasting pan. Sprinkle the paprika over the potatoes and mix well to coat. Roast on the bottom rack 1 hour 10 minutes, turning several times during cooking, or until tender. Serves 6.

PER SERVING: ⅙ of recipe

2½ 🔲

Calories	176
g protein	4
g carbohydrate	41
g dietary fiber	3
g fat–total	0
g saturated fat	0
mg cholesterol	0
mg sodium	98

Mince Tarts

Use a small star or holly cutter to decorate the mince tarts. I always make my pastry in a food processor, which gives a shorter texture and makes handling easier.

1	recipe Pastry for Normandy Apple Flan (page 161)	1
¼ cup	Meatless Mincemeat (page 173)	60 mL
	A little milk for glazing	
	A little granulated artificial sweetener (optional)	

❖ Suitable for freezing. Cool and pack into a rigid freezer container. Freeze up to three months. Thaw and then warm in a hot oven 3 to 4 minutes before serving.

Prepare and chill the pastry as directed on page 161.

Preheat oven to 400°F (200°C). Roll pastry out on a lightly floured board. Using a 2½-inch (6-cm) round cutter and a small star cutter, cut out an equal number of rounds and stars.

Place the pastry rounds in mini muffin cups or small tart pans. Add 1 tsp (5 mL) of mincemeat to each. Place a star on mincemeat in each tart. Bake 10 to 15 minutes or until crust is golden brown. Brush with a little milk and sprinkle with a little sweetener if desired when the pies come out of the oven. Serve warm. Makes 12 to 16 tarts.

PER SERVING: ½ of recipe

½ ☐ + ½ ◪ + 1 ◭

Calories	111
g protein	2
g carbohydrate	14
g dietary fiber	1
g fat–total	5
g saturated fat	1
mg cholesterol	0
mg sodium	72

Sangria

This will remind you of hot sunny holidays in Mexico!

1	bottle nonalcoholic red wine	750 mL
1½ cups	unsweetened orange juice	375 mL
1	1-quart (1 L) bottle diet lemonade	1
	A few orange slices	
	Ice cubes	

Mix the wine, orange juice and lemonade together in a large pitcher or punch bowl. Add the orange slices and ice. Serve chilled. Makes 10 servings.

PER SERVING: ¹⁄₁₀ of recipe

Calories	39
g protein	1
g carbohydrate	9
g dietary fiber	0
g fat–total	0
g saturated fat	0
mg cholesterol	0
mg sodium	8

Frozen Fruit Bombe

This dessert makes a delicious and refreshing alternative to a rich dessert.

1	envelope unflavored gelatin	1
½ cup	water	125 mL
1	6-oz (175 mL) can evaporated milk, chilled overnight	1
1	8-oz (250 g) carton light cream cheese, softened	1
1 tbsp	granulated artificial sweetener	15 mL
¾ cup	dark raisins	175 mL
2 tbsp	brandy	25 mL
¼ cup	slivered almonds	60 mL

Combine gelatin and water in a small saucepan. Let stand 5 minutes to soften gelatin. Heat over low heat, stirring, until gelatin dissolves. Set aside to cool. Whisk the evaporated milk in a chilled bowl until double in size and stiff peaks form. Fold the cooled gelatin into the evaporated milk together with the cheese and sweetener. Place in a shallow tray and freeze 1 hour or until partially set. Soak the raisins in the brandy.

Turn milk mixture into a bowl and whisk thoroughly. Stir in the almonds and soaked raisins. Place in a lightly greased 1-quart (1-L) metal bowl. Freeze overnight or until solid. Remove from the freezer 5 minutes before serving. Turn out on to a serving plate and serve immediately. Makes 6 servings.

PER SERVING: ⅙ of recipe

2 ◼ + ½ ◆ Whole
+ ½ ◩ + 2½ ▲

Calories	250
g protein	9
g carbohydrate	23
g dietary fiber	1
g fat–total	15
g saturated fat	6
mg cholesterol	35
mg sodium	327

Fruit Cake

Small servings of this special-occasion cake are perfect for Christmas.

1 cup	all-purpose flour	250 mL
1 tsp	baking soda	5 mL
½ tsp	salt	2 mL
1 tsp	ground cinnamon	5 mL
1 tsp	mixed spice	5 mL
½ tsp	grated nutmeg	2 mL
8 oz	raisins	250 g
8 oz	currants	250 g
8 oz	golden raisins	250 g
4 oz	glacé cherries, rinsed, dried and quartered	120 g
4 oz	slivered almonds	120 g
½ cup	soft margarine	125 mL
¼ cup	packed brown sugar	60 mL
4	eggs, beaten	4
3 tbsp	brandy	50 mL

Preheat oven to 300°F (150°C). Grease and line a heavy 8-inch (20-cm) round or square cake pan with a double thickness of waxed paper.

Sift together the flour, baking soda, salt and spices, adding back any bran remaining in the sifter. Mix together the fruit and almonds. Beat the margarine and sugar together until pale and creamy. Gradually beat in the eggs, adding a tbsp of flour mixture with each egg. Fold in the remaining flour, fruit and brandy.

Spoon the mixture into the prepared pan and level the surface. Make a slight well in the center with the back of a spoon. Bake about 2½ hours or until a skewer inserted in the center comes out clean. Cover the cake with foil if it browns too quickly. Cool in the pan 30 minutes. Turn out on to a wire rack, remove the paper and allow to cool completely. Wrap well and store in a cool place. Makes 32 servings.

PER SERVING: ⅟₃₂ of recipe

2 ▰ + ½ ✳ + 1 ◮

Calories	151
g protein	3
g carbohydrate	24
g dietary fiber	1
g fat–total	5
g saturated fat	1
mg cholesterol	27
mg sodium	110

Meatless Mincemeat

Making your own mincemeat means that you can cut down on the sugar content considerably. This recipe has a natural sweetness from just the dried fruit and fruit juice. However, it will need to be used within one week or frozen in a plastic container for up to three months.

❖ Use to make Mince Tarts (page 169).

8 oz	raisins	250 g
8 oz	golden raisins	250 g
4 oz	dried apricots, finely chopped	120 g
4 oz	glacé cherries, rinsed, dried and finely chopped	120 g
2 oz	chopped mixed nuts	60 g
1	large carrot, peeled and finely grated	1
	Finely grated peel and juice of 1 lemon	
¼ cup	unsweetened orange juice	60 mL
1 tbsp	brandy or rum (optional)	15 mL

Mix all the ingredients together in a large bowl. Cover and refrigerate 2 days, stirring occasionally.

Use as desired or pack into clean, sterilized jars and refrigerate up to 1 week or freeze in plastic containers up to 3 months. Makes about 2 lb (1 kg).

PER SERVING: ¹⁄₁₀ of recipe

4 ▱ + 1 ✳ + ½ ◮

Calories	239
g protein	3
g carbohydrate	55
g dietary fiber	3
g fat–total	3
g saturated fat	0
mg cholesterol	0
mg sodium	10

Index

• *Italicized text indicates sidebar material*

ALMOND
    Lemon and Almond Cake, 125
    Spiced Apple and Almond Cake, 122
APPLE
    Apple and Blackberry Sponge Pudding, 140
    Apple Pie in Walnut Pastry, 133
    Normandy Apple Flan, 161–62
    Rice Pudding with Apple and Blackberry, 144
    Sautéed Pork with Apple, 68
    Spiced Apple and Almond Cake, 122
    Spiced Apple Pie in Filo Pastry, 145
    Steamed Apple and Berry Pudding, 143
APRICOTS
    Apricot and Raisin Bread, 106
    Apricot-Pecan Loaf, 102
    Apricot Upside-Down Cake, 118
    Chickpea, Apricot and Cashew Pilaf, 51
    Date and Apricot Bars, 127
    Pork and Apricot Casserole, 67
ASPARAGUS
    Flaky Salmon and Asparagus Tart, 41

BANANAS
    Banana Bread, 100
    Banana Cream Pie, 139
    Carrot and Banana Cake, 114
BASIL
    Red Pepper, Basil and Tuna Pasta Salad, 28
Beans. *See* Peas, Beans, Legumes
BEEF
    Beef and Lentil Hot Pot, 61
    Beef Burgundy, 66
    Beef Casserole with Herb Dumplings, 60
    Beef, Pepper and Baby Corn Stir-Fry, 65
    Cheesy Shepherd's Pie, 71
    Light Pastitsio, 63–64
    Peppered Roast Beef, 160
    Spicy Hungarian Goulash, 70
BERRIES
    Apple and Blackberry Sponge Pudding, 140
    Chocolate and Strawberry Roll, 115
    Cranberry Sauce, 158
    Figs with Blackberry Sauce, 146
    Nectarine and Raspberry Dessert, 150
    Peach and Raspberry Rice, 144
    Pears with Raspberry Sauce, 141
    Raspberry Trifle, 164
    Rice Pudding with Apple and Blackberry, 144
    Steamed Apple and Berry Pudding, 143
    Strawberry Creams, 136
    Strawberry Milkshake, 155
BEVERAGES
    Peach Melba Shake, 155
    Sangria, 170
    Strawberry Milkshake, 155
BREADS and MUFFINS
    Apricot and Raisin Bread, 106
    Apricot-Pecan Loaf, 102
    Banana Bread, 100
    Buttermilk Cornbread, 99
    Cheese and Bacon Bread, 108
    Cherry and Walnut Bread, 107
    Farmhouse Fruit Scones, 104
    Ginger and Date Bread, 105
    Granary Loaf, 110
    Herb and Garlic Bread, 18
    Hot Cross Buns, 111
    Lemon-Sesame Bread, 103
    Low-Fat Garlic Croutons, 15
    Raisin-Nut Muffins, 101
    Whole-Wheat Bread, 109

Cajun seasoning, 77
CAKES and COOKIES
    Apricot-Pecan Loaf, 102
    Apricot Upside-Down Cake, 118
    Baking-Powder Biscuits, 98
    Carrot and Banana Cake, 114
    Cherry and Raisin Cake, 121
    Chocolate and Strawberry Roll, 115
    Chocolate Squares, 120
    Coconut and Cherry Fingers, 119
    Date and Apricot Bars, 127
    Fruit Cake, 172
    German Plum Coffeecake, 123
    Lemon Cake, 124
    Orange and Ginger Cookies, 126
    Pinolata, 117
    Raisin Cookies, 128
    Spiced Apple and Almond Cake, 122
    Spiced Mandarin Gâteau, 116
    Tropical Island Cookies, 129
    Yellow Cake, 130
CARROTS
    Carrot and Banana Cake, 114
    Lentil and Root Vegetable Hot Pot, 55
CHEESE
    Cheese and Bacon Bread, 108
    Cheese and Spinach Filo Triangles, 23
    Cheesy Shepherd's Pie, 71
    Endive Gratin, 72
    Fresh Leek Soup with Blue Cheese, 11
    Lemon and Raisin Cheesecake, 134
    Lime Torte, 152
    Mediterranean Gougère, 45–46
    Pineapple and Lemon Cheesecake, 135
CHERRIES
    Cherry and Raisin Cake, 121
    Cherry and Walnut Bread, 107
    Clafouti, 153
    Coconut and Cherry Fingers, 119

CHICKEN
    Catalonian Chicken, 80
    Chicken Marengo, 78
    Chicken-Sausage Sauce, 92
    Chicken, Spicy Sausage and Seafood Paella, 73
    Chicken Tikka, 82
    Georgia Chicken, 77
    Marinated Chicken and Rosemary Kebabs, 74
    Mushroom and Chicken Tagliatelle, 88
    Spiced Chicken Brochettes with Couscous, Red Bean and Coriander Pilaf, 75–76
    Spicy Chicken Satay with Creamy Peanut Dip, 17
    Traditional Roast Chicken with Raisin and Parsley Stuffing, 83
CHILE
    Monkfish, Tiger Prawn and Chile Stir-Fry, 34
CHOCOLATE
    Chocolate and Strawberry Roll, 115
    Chocolate Squares, 120
CILANTRO
    Fish with Ginger and Cilantro, 26
COCONUT
    Coconut and Cherry Fingers, 119
    Spicy Tomato and Coconut Fish Curry, 29
CORIANDER
    Spiced Chicken Brochettes with Couscous, Red Bean and Coriander Pilaf, 75–76
CORN
    Beef, Pepper and Baby Corn Stir-Fry, 65
    Corn and Salmon Cakes with Yogurt-Herb Dressing, 32
    Sweet Pepper, Baby Corn and Smoked Fish Stir-Fry, 38
Cornbread, 99
CORNISH HENS
    Roast Rock Cornish Hens, 159
    Rock Cornish Hens, 81
COUSCOUS
    Spiced Chicken Brochettes with Couscous, Red Bean and Coriander Pilaf, 75–76
CURRY
    Creamy Curried Potato Salad, 57
    Eastern Spiced Vegetables, 58
    Lamb Rhogan, 69
    Spicy Tomato and Coconut Fish Curry, 29

DATES
    Date and Apricot Bars, 127
    Ginger and Date Bread, 105
DESSERTS
    (*See also* Cakes and Cookies; Pies)
    Apple and Blackberry Sponge Pudding, 140
    Apricot-Pecan Loaf, 102
    Chilled Lemon Soufflé, 147

Clafouti, 153
Creamy Fruit Dessert, 166
Figs with Blackberry Sauce, 146
Frozen Fruit Bombe, 171
Frozen Orange Cups, 151
Lime Torte, 152
Nectarine and Raspberry Dessert, 150
No-Added-Sugar Steamed Pudding, 165
Normandy Apple Flan, 161–62
Old-Fashioned Baked Custard Tart, 132
Peach and Raspberry Rice, 144
Peach Yogurt Crunch, 154
Pears with Raspberry Sauce, 141
Plum Sponge Pudding, 140
Rhubarb and Ginger Fool, 137
Rice Pudding with Apple and Blackberry, 144
Steamed Apple and Berry Pudding, 143
Strawberry Creams, 136
Strawberry Milkshake, 155
Summer Fruit Layers, 142
Tiramisu, 158
Tropical Paradise Fruit Salad, 163
DIPS and SPREADS
Crispy Potato Skins with Tomato and Yogurt Dips, 19
Quick and Easy Sardine Pâté, 22
Quick Chickpea Dip, 12
Quick Tomato Salsa, 14
Spicy Chicken Satay with Creamy Peanut Dip, 17
Dumplings, 60

EGGS
Chilled Lemon Soufflé, 147
Fresh Herb and Shrimp Omelet, 42
Mexican Black-Eyed Pea and Spinach Omelet, 50
Mini Yorkshire Puddings, 167
Old-Fashioned Baked Custard Tart, 132
ENDIVE
Endive Gratin, 72

Feta cheese, 47
FIGS
Figs with Blackberry Sauce, 146
Filo pastry, 36
FISH
(See also Seafood)
Baked Fresh Salmon and Spinach in Light Pastry, 33
Baked Mushroom and Cod Crumble, 27
Baked Zucchini, Red Pepper and Tuna Pasta, 89
Broiled Salmon with Garlic and Peppercorns, 39
Corn and Salmon Cakes with Yogurt-Herb Dressing, 32
Fish with Ginger and Cilantro, 26
Fishermen's Crispy Filo Pie, 36–37
Flaky Salmon and Asparagus Tart, 41
Light Salad Niçoise, 49

Monkfish, Tiger Prawn and Chile Stir-Fry, 34
Quick and Easy Sardine Pâté, 22
Red Pepper, Basil and Tuna Pasta Salad, 28
Seafood Lasagna, 87
Spicy Tomato and Coconut Fish Curry, 29
Sweet Pepper, Baby Corn and Smoked Fish Stir-Fry, 38
Szechwan Fish Pie, 40
Watercress-and-Smoked-Salmon Roll, 24
Zesty Lemon Fish in Packages, 35
FRUIT
Chilled Fruit-Filled Melon, 21
Creamy Fruit Dessert, 166
Farmhouse Fruit Scones, 104
Frozen Fruit Bombe, 171
Fruit Cake, 172
Summer Fruit Layers, 142
Tropical Paradise Fruit Salad, 163

Garam masala, 29
GARLIC
Broiled Salmon with Garlic and Peppercorns, 39
Herb and Garlic Bread, 18
Low-fat Garlic Croutons, 15
Gelatin, 135
GINGER, 26
Fish with Ginger and Cilantro, 26
Ginger and Date Bread, 105
Orange and Ginger Cookies, 126
Rhubarb and Ginger Fool, 137

HAM
Creamy Leek and Ham Tart, 62
Endive Gratin, 72
Ham and Tomato Pasta Sauce, 90
HERBS
Beef Casserole with Herb Dumplings, 60
Corn and Salmon Cakes with Yogurt-Herb Dressing, 32
Fresh Herb and Shrimp Omelet, 32
Herb and Garlic Bread, 18
Hot pot(s), 61

JELLY
Creamy Fruit Dessert, 166
Raspberry Trifle, 164
Strawberry Creams, 136
Summer Fruit Layers, 142

LAMB
Lamb Rhogan, 69
LEEKS, 11
Creamy Leak and Ham Tart, 62
LEMON
Chilled Lemon Soufflé, 147
Lemon and Almond Cake, 125
Lemon and Lime Meringue Pie, 149
Lemon and Raisin Cheesecake, 134
Lemon Cake, 124
Lemon-Sesame Bread, 103

Pineapple and Lemon Cheesecake, 135
Zesty Lemon Fish in Packages, 35
LIME
Lemon and Lime Meringue Pie, 149
Lime Torte, 152

MILK
Buttermilk Cornbread, 99
Strawberry Milkshake, 155
MUSHROOMS
Baked Mushroom and Cod Crumble, 27
Chicken Marengo, 78
Flageolet Bean and Mushroom Korma, 52
Mushroom and Chicken Tagliatelle, 88

NECTARINES
Nectarine and Raspberry Dessert, 150
NUTS and SEEDS
Apple Pie in Walnut Pastry, 133
Apricot-Pecan Loaf, 102
Cherry and Walnut Bread, 107
Chickpea, Apricot and Cashew Pilaf, 51
Lemon-Sesame Bread, 103
Rock Cornish Hens with Walnuts, 79
Spaghetti Tossed with Turkey and Walnuts, 86
Spicy Chicken Satay with Creamy Peanut Dip, 17

OMELETS
Fresh Herb and Shrimp Omelet, 42
Mexican Black-Eyed Pea and Spinach Omelet, 50
ONIONS
Tomato and Red Onion Salad, 48
ORANGES
Frozen Orange Cups, 151
Mandarin Creams, 136
Orange and Ginger Cookies, 126
Spiced Mandarin Gâteau, 116

PARSLEY
Parsley Croquettes, 19
Traditional Roast Chicken with Raisin and Parsley Stuffing, 83
PASTA, 63
Baked Zucchini, Red Pepper and Tuna Pasta, 89
Italian Red Bean and Pasta Soup, 13
Light Pastitsio, 63
Mushroom and Chicken Tagliatelle, 88
Red Pepper, Basil and Tuna Pasta Salad, 28
Red Pesto Pasta, 94
Sauce (Ham and Tomato), 90
Seafood Lasagna, 87
Spaghetti Tossed with Turkey and Walnuts, 86
Stir-Fried Shredded Pork and Pasta, 91
Ten-Minute Carbonara, 93
PASTRY
(See also Pies)
Apple Pie in Walnut Pastry, 133

Baked Fresh Salmon and Spinach in Light Pastry, 33
Cheese and Spinach Filo Triangles, 23
Creamy Crab and Red Pepper Tart, 30
Creamy Leak and Ham Tart, 62
Fishermen's Crispy Filo, 36
Flaky Salmon and Asparagus Tart, 41
Mediterranean Gougère, 45
Mince Tarts, 169
Normandy Apple Flan, 161–62
Sweet Spiced Apple Pie in Filo Pastry, 145
Szechwan Fish Pie, 40
PEACHES
Peach and Raspberry Rice, 144
Peach Melba Shake, 155
Peach Yogurt Crunch, 154
PEARS
Pears with Raspberry Sauce, 141
PEAS, BEANS, LEGUMES, 11, 13, 67
Beef and Lentil Hot Pot, 61
Black-Eyed Pea and Vegetable Soup, 10
Black-Eyed Pea Crumble, 54
Chickpea, Apricot and Cashew Pilaf, 51
Cowboy's Supper, 84
Easy Green and Red Bean Salad, 44
Flageolet Bean and Mushroom Korma, 52
Italian Red Bean and Pasta Soup, 13
Lentil and Root Vegetable Hot Pot, 55
Mexican Black-Eyed Pea and Spinach Omelet, 50
Quick Chickpea Dip, 12
Spiced Chicken Brochettes with Couscous, Red Bean and Coriander Pilaf, 75–76
Yellow Split-Pea and Turkey Sauce, 95
PESTO
Red Pesto Pasta, 94
PIES and TARTS
Apple Pie in Walnut Pastry, 133
Banana Cream Pie, 139
Lemon and Lime Meringue Pie, 149
Mince Tarts, 169
Meatless Mincemeat, 173
Spiced Apple Pie in Filo Pastry, 145
Pilaf, 75
Pine nuts, 117
PINEAPPLE, 163
Pineapple and Lemon Cheesecake, 135
Pinto beans, 67
PLUMS
German Plum Coffeecake, 123
Plum Sponge Pudding, 140
PORK
Pork and Apricot Casserole, 67
Sautéed Pork with Apple, 68
Stir-Fried Shredded Pork and Pasta, 91
POTATOES
Creamy Curried Potato Salad, 57
Crispy Potato Skins with Tomato and Yogurt Dips, 19
Dry-Roasted Potatoes, 168
Parsley Croquettes, 19

RAISINS
Apricot and Raisin Bread, 106
Cherry and Raisin Cake, 121
Lemon and Raisin Cheesecake, 134
Raisin Cookies, 128
Raisin-Nut Muffins, 101
Traditional Roast Chicken with Raisin and Parsley Stuffing, 83
RED PEPPERS
Baked Zucchini, Red Pepper and Tuna Pasta, 89
Beef, Pepper and Baby Corn Stir-Fry, 65
Creamy Crab and Red Pepper Tart, 30
Red Pepper, Basil and Tuna Pasta Salad, 28
Sweet Pepper, Baby Corn and Smoked Fish Stir-Fry, 38
RHUBARB
Rhubarb and Ginger Fool, 137
RICE
Chickpea, Apricot and Cashew Pilaf, 51
Peach and Raspberry Rice, 144
Rice Pudding with Apple and Blackberry, 144
Risotto Primavera, 56
ROSEMARY
Marinated Chicken and Rosemary Kebabs, 74

SALADS
Creamy Curried Potato Salad, 57
Easy Green and Red Bean Salad, 44
Greek Salad, 47
Light Salad Niçoise, 49
Red Pepper, Basil and Tuna Pasta Salad, 28
Tomato and Red Onion Salad, 48
Tropical Paradise Fruit Salad, 163
Sangria, 170
SAUCES
Chicken-Sausage Sauce, 92
Cranberry Sauce, 158
Figs with Blackberry Sauce, 146
Ham and Tomato Pasta Sauce, 90
No-Sugar Custard Sauce, 148
Raspberry Sauce, 141
Yellow Split-Pea and Turkey Sauce, 95
SAUSAGES
Chicken-Sausage Sauce, 92
Chicken, Spicy Sausage and Seafood Paella, 73
Cowboy's Supper, 84
SEAFOOD
Chicken, Spicy Sausage and Seafood Paella, 73
Creamy Crab and Red Pepper Tart, 30
Fresh Herb and Shrimp Omelet, 42
Monkfish, Tiger Prawn and Chile Stir-Fry, 34
Seafood Lasagna, 87
Tiger Prawn Jambalaya, 31
SOUPS
Black-Eyed Pea and Vegetable Soup, 10

Chilled Summer Gazpacho, 15
Fresh Leek Soup with Blue Cheese, 11
Hearty Winter Vegetable Soup, 20
Italian Red Bean and Pasta Soup, 13
Spicy Winter Mulligatawny, 16
SPINACH
Baked Fresh Salmon and Spinach in Light Pastry, 33
Cheese and Spinach Filo Triangles, 23
Mexican Black-Eyed Pea and Spinach Omelet, 50
STUFFING
Traditional Roast Chicken with Raisin and Parsley Stuffing, 83
Tiger prawns, 31
TOMATOES
Chicken Marengo, 78
Crispy Potato Skins with Tomato and Yogurt Dips, 19
Ham and Tomato Pasta Sauce, 90
Quick Tomato Salsa, 14
Spicy Tomato and Coconut Fish Curry, 29
Tomato and Red Onion Salad, 48
TURKEY
Spaghetti Tossed with Turkey and Walnuts, 86
Yellow Split-Pea and Turkey Sauce, 95
VEGETABLES
Black-Eyed Pea and Vegetable Soup, 10
Chilled Summer Gazpacho, 15
Eastern Spiced Vegetables, 58
Hearty Winter Vegetable Soup, 20
Lentil and Root Vegetable Hot Pot, 55
Mediterranean Gougère, 45
Risotto Primavera, 56
Spicy Cajun Casserole, 53
Vegetable Thatch Pie, 71
WATERCRESS
Watercress-and-Smoked-Salmon Roll, 24
YOGURT
Corn and Salmon Cakes with Yogurt-Herb Dressing, 32
Crispy Potato Skins with Tomato and Yogurt Dips, 19
Peach Melba Shake, 155
Peach Yogurt Crunch, 154
Strawberry Milkshake, 155
Yorkshire Pudding, 167
ZUCCHINI
Baked Zucchini, Red Pepper and Tuna Pasta, 89